From Chunk to Hunk
Diary of a Fat Man

three toes publishing

From Chunk to Hunk
Diary of a Fat Man

by Fred Anderson

Published by:

Three Toes Publishing
PO Box 565
Madison, AL 35758 USA

ISBN 0-9741500-0-2

First printing August 2003

Printed in the United States of America

From Chunk to Hunk
Diary of a Fat Man

Fred Anderson

for the naysayers

Introduction

371 – 341 *pounds*

I wasn't *always* fat.

As a child I was only a little overweight – not even big enough to wear the husky size. When I first started paying attention to my size at fourteen I weighed 156, about 15 pounds too much. By the time I graduated high school three and a half years later, I was hovering at about 200 pounds.

When I graduated from college in 1990 I was up to 260 pounds, with apparently no upper limit in sight. As a desk jockey writing computer software, I blossomed to 330 pounds before I made my first serious attempt to lose weight. I lost 50 pounds in two months by starving myself on about 1000 calories a day just to impress a girl I was dating, and promptly gained it back when we broke up. Shortly afterward, I met my future wife, Robyn, and within a year my weight crept up to a looming 371 pounds.

It gets worse. Even though I was diagnosed with adult-onset diabetes in 1997, I didn't really do anything about my weight. My doctor put me on increasing amounts of medication to help my body use the insulin it produced (my diabetes was caused by a condition called insulin resistance, which means, in a nutshell, that there was so much fat in me that my body couldn't use its own insulin to clear the glucose from my blood) but it didn't really help me at all. Why? I loved food, plain and simple, and I especially loved sweet foods. From cookies to cakes and everything in between, I could never get enough. I'd eat things like white bread with sugar and butter on it for a snack, and in a pinch I'd even eat sugar out of the bag.

My daily eating pattern was to skip breakfast, have a big lunch from one of the numerous restaurants near my office, some kind of snack when

I got home from work, then stuff myself with things like pot roast and mashed potatoes with gravy at dinnertime. The high point of the day – my favorite time – came after dinner. Snack-time, I called it.

Yeah, right. Like three or four Little Debbie snack cakes is a snack; or a whole pint of Ben and Jerry's ice cream; or half a bag of Oreo cookies. And I wondered, like an idiot, why my doctor kept increasing my diabetes medicine when she would check my blood sugar.

Thank God for reality television.

When you're fat it is easy to pretend that you aren't, to pretend that you are just another person walking down the street without a care in the world. You don't forget how fat you are, but you successfully block it from your conscious mind. Sometimes, however, you get a harsh reminder. Mine came over my birthday weekend in May 2000, when my wife Robyn and I took our daughter, Danielle, on a vacation to the Smoky Mountains. That was where my wakeup call began.

Danielle wanted to ride a virtual roller coaster and I climbed in with her. Halfway through, I had to stop the ride because I was terrified the seatbelt holding me in was going to snap during one of the numerous times the machine suspended us upside-down. With my 370+ pounds and her 130, we were a good twenty pounds over the machine's posted weight limit of 480 pounds.

We also tried the Ripley's Motion Theater, which is like a normal movie house except the seats move – and they move violently. I was so big I had to force my frame into the seat, and to hold on I used the handgrips in the seats on either side of me. The seatbelt barely made it around my gut, and my arms got bruised all over because they were outside my seat and banged on other seats.

I learned a valuable lesson from those two rides. Can you imagine what it feels like to tell your child that you cannot share a ride with her because you are afraid you won't fit, or that you are concerned you'll break it?

We returned home the Sunday before Memorial Day. After three and a half days of walking in one-block stretches because I couldn't go any further without resting my aching feet and knees, all I wanted when I got home was some good TV time with my sweet snacks. As it turns out, I got exactly what I needed.

I settled onto the couch with a Little Debbie strawberry shortcake roll. Before I started eating, I spent several minutes surfing channels looking for something to entertain me while I ate, because really, isn't mindless eating the best kind of eating? I settled on an emergency room documentary.

In this particular show, a middle-aged man lay in the emergency room complaining about a bad pain in one of his feet, which was wrapped in a towel. According to the doctor narrating the story, he was a diabetic and he didn't take care of his disease. As I took my first bite of the strawberry roll the man unwrapped his foot, revealing several crusty black rotten toes and a foot covered with suppurating sores. His leg had to be amputated right below the knee. While the amputation wasn't shown, what was shown was worse: the man moaning and crying when the doctor told him that his leg would have to go.

In that man's story I saw my own story, and what the not too distant future had in store for me. I didn't like what I saw, and resolved that something had to change.

I got off the couch and threw away the rest of the strawberry roll. The thought of having my own leg amputated was enough to *instantly* transform the way I viewed what I was eating.

I can still imagine, at times, what Ebenezer Scrooge must have felt when he realized it was still Christmas morning and the future of his dream had not yet come to pass. That moment awakened me from a deep sleep, and showed me that the time had come to get my act together. I went cold turkey on the sweet foods, and within a week I was working out doing the only thing I was physically able to do: treading water for 10 minutes at a time.

A couple of weeks later I had to visit my doctor because I was almost out of my diabetes medicine, and it was time to go through my humiliating quarterly blood tests. My doctor believed very strongly in the carrot and stick philosophy, and as a result, wrote my prescriptions such that I had to go back to see her every three months.

Normally, I argued with the head nurse about weighing, because it's pretty painful to slide the weights all the way to their heaviest setting only to find that it's still not enough to accurately depict my weight. *This time*, I thought to myself, *maybe my eating and treading water for these last two weeks has done some good.* I stepped up onto the scales, holding my breath.

I weighed 347 pounds.

While I was there that day, in addition to performing the normal hemoglobin A1c test, which measures the average amount of glucose in your blood over a three-month period, she also did a fructosamine test and checked my blood sugar. While my hemoglobin A1c showed me a little high – after all, it does measure three months' worth of sugar effects, and I'd only started to change myself a couple of weeks ago – the other two were already in the perfectly normal range.

I felt better those first days than I had in the last several years. I had more energy, and I didn't have to take a nap every day after work just to recover from the hard job of sitting at a desk. Throughout these days, I ate less food than I'd previously consumed, I avoided sugar, and I treaded water. My blood sugar was staying between 90 and 100 (normal is considered to be anything between 70 and 110). Two weeks of doing something I should have been doing all along, coupled with the diabetes pills, brought my blood sugar into the normal range.

I went by my doctor's office again a week later just to weigh. Talk about change – the man who used to hide from the scales or proclaim that he would just "skip this part" when asked to weigh was now making special trips to the doctor's office just to be weighed. The result? 341 pounds. I was pumped.

Almost three years and over 170 pounds later, I'm still pumped. This book, originally my personal journal, is the end result of that process. I used my journal to document the path I took, to share my thoughts and ideas in hopes that it would reach others trapped in a world of fat like I was, and show them that a dramatic physical transformation is possible without diets, pills, or surgery.

I didn't actually start writing in the journal until I weighed 341 pounds, thirty pounds below my highest weight. I began writing near the end of June 2000, and continued to write for over two years. During those two years as I transformed physically, I also transformed mentally.

For example, I was concerned in the beginning mostly with simply eating less food, while still eating many of the processed (i.e., junk) foods I once ate, sweets notwithstanding. As I learned more about nutrition, my opinions about food changed, and as a result, the foods I now eat are mostly unprocessed. Because of this gradual mental transformation, this book might not make sense if you sit down and read it from cover to cover in one sitting. Read it in small pieces, and take the time to consider the points I discuss. Think about how you can use them to transform yourself. Use them, and watch yourself become the person you've always wanted to be.

June 2000

341 – 335 pounds

June 25

I'm not particularly concerned with my caloric intake. I'm not on a diet because I believe diets don't work, at least not for someone as big as me. Someone my size needs a whole new way of eating, something designed to last the rest of his life.

I'm simply eating healthier food. As someone who needs to watch his blood sugar, I try to keep my carbohydrates per meal to around 60 or 70 grams. My doctor tells me that once I lose my weight, I won't have to be so careful about watching carbohydrates, because my body will be using its insulin properly. When she diagnosed me with diabetes in 1997 my doctor gave me an 1800-calorie diet, but the dietician she sent me to said I would starve on it and that I should be eating about 2500 calories per day. I'm not sure which to believe, so I just eat what seems right.

Life's too short to spend my time weighing and measuring what I eat.

My body knows when it has had enough, and it can tell me better than either my doctor or a dietician. I got this fat through a combination of eating too much and moving too little. Instead of eating until I'm stuffed, now I merely eat until I'm full. I'm eating more vegetables every day, and several pieces of fruit. The change in my energy level is astounding.

I've tried to lose weight before, from various drinkable diets in the 80's to pills in the 90's to the more recent fad diets sweeping the nation. None of them worked for me. Not because I don't have willpower (more on that later), but because I hadn't made the decision to change my weight permanently.

It's all about your decisions, I've found.

You decide what you're going to put in your mouth and you decide whether or not you're going to move your body. The root of the word "decide" is from Middle French and Latin, and means literally "to cut off." What I needed to do before I could begin my life-changing weight loss was to make a decision, to cut off any other option. I did this through the help of a good mental anchor: seeing a diabetic man with a rotting foot that had to be amputated. That was my wake up call, and I don't plan on going back to sleep any time soon.

June 26

Most diets don't make sense, under scrutiny. Look at the whole idea behind Slim-Fast. What kind of person can just stop eating two of their three daily meals, and substitute a glass of what is basically sugared water for those meals? If you're like most people, the minute you come off the plan, you start gaining weight again.

Look at the "success stories" on the Slim-Fast web page, or watch one of their commercials. Examine it closely and you'll see a disclaimer: "Results not typical." Even the manufacturer knows that people have a tendency to gain the weight back after they starve it off. I'm not accusing them of false advertising, I just want to point out that people cannot effectively lose weight and keep it off without something more than a "diet."

I'm not a religious person, but I've studied the Bible extensively, and if I may paraphrase the Apostle Paul: "All things in moderation." Sugar is not unhealthy in and of itself, but the abuse of sugar – something I once did, with bags of cookies and pounds of candy bars – is indeed unhealthy. Everyone knows water is necessary for sustaining life. However, too much water and you can develop a condition called water intoxication, which makes you dizzy, confused and can lead to a coma or even death. Exercise your brain when you eat; a little common sense goes a long way.

For me, the key to losing weight is not about depriving myself of anything. A question for you: what's the basic human instinct when we think there's something we cannot have?

We want it even more! That leads to bingeing, for example, and is a big factor in failed diets. Today's fad diets involve a radical deprivation of some sort, and are ultimately doomed to fail for most people. The key is changing your eating habits by changing your mental associations with food.

June 27

People have many powerful mental associations with food. For some, eating may be associated with guilt: remember those starving kids in China your mom warned you about? For others, there may be a sense of reward: clean your plate and you can have some ice cream!

For still others – and this was my problem – food was pleasure at its basest level. I immersed myself in my eating. I particularly enjoyed sweet foods like cakes, cookies, and candies. The sight of them made me weak, and I'd do anything to just eat, and eat, and eat. My epiphany changed that, and enabled me to completely re-associate the sight of sugary foods with complications arising from diabetes.

The new association is so strong it's almost humorous. A co-worker at my job also owns part of a local cinnamon roll shop, and he periodically brings in a big bag of nice warm, gooey, rolls. I used to help him eat them, but not anymore. He brought some in yesterday, and while my office manager helped herself to one as we talked in the break area, she said, "I guess I shouldn't eat these in front of you so I don't tempt you."

According to the dictionary, the word "disgust" means "to excite nausea or loathing in; sicken." What my office manager doesn't understand is that when I look at the pile of cinnamon rolls, all I can see is a gangrenous festering foot. The buttery sugar glaze reminds me of running pus, and the pecans on the top are like little maggots feasting on the decay. The cinnamon smell seems a little rancid to me and it's not too hard to imagine that I'm not only seeing the foot, but smelling it too. It's that visceral to me.

Do I want one? You've got to be kidding.

Besides sweet foods, my other big downfall was fatty cuts of red meat, particularly steaks with a good ring of fat around the edge. No longer. Have you ever watched heart bypass surgery on TV? The doctor cuts open the artery to reveal something white, cheesy, and crusty. He grabs it and slowly pulls it out, twisting it back and forth because it is wedged so tightly in the artery. When completely removed, the blockage can reach a length of up to two feet, and looks kind of the way bacon grease does when you put it in the fridge.

Another method I use is to imagine a plateful of something I want, but with an extra ingredient or two thrown in for good measure. Vomit and feces seem to work best for me.

These are just a couple of the things I use to change my associations with certain foods. Using offensive and disgusting images is not the only way to change your associations to foods. As a matter of fact, I use positive reinforcements much more often than negative ones. As far as I'm concerned, the only time to bring out the disgust is when I feel like I'm in real danger.

One thing that brings me total pleasure now is the knowledge that what I'm eating is healthful and that it fortifies my body. I eat loads of vegetables and a goodly amount of fruit, though I have to be mindful of the fruit, thanks to the diabetes. When I pick up either of these, I form images in my head of the vitamins and minerals literally bursting out of the food , going to work to help my body rejuvenate and be nourished. Hokey, but it works.

A question I like to ask myself before I eat anything is: "Will this food help me or hurt me?" If a food will help my health, I eat it. If I believe the food will hurt me, I generally don't. We know which foods are healthy, and which aren't. We're not stupid. No one knows as well as a fat person which foods are healthy and which foods aren't.

June 28

Humans have two basic mental and physical motivators. We do things that bring us pleasure and we avoid things that bring us pain. I was discussing this idea with a friend yesterday and he asked me the following: "How do you encourage yourself to move towards the pleasure of having lost so much weight while having the pain (discouragement, hunger, plateaus) the path to your goal brings?"

In losing weight, perspective is everything. As such, I don't view this path as painful. In my mind, the goal is the very epitome of pleasure. At that weight I can do anything I want. I won't have to worry about not fitting into the seats of carnival rides, or being breathless from walking up a flight of stairs. I'll be able to do things with my wife and our daughter without having to stop and rest. I can shop in normal clothing stores without being labeled "big" anymore. As much energy as I have after dropping only 35 pounds, how much more will I have when I lose the rest?

Each time I eat a piece of food that takes me closer to that goal, I feel pleasure. Each time I climb onto my stationary bike, I'm happy. (Except for my butt, which hasn't gotten used to the seat.) When I swim I'm ecstatic, because I'm creating my dream and achieving my goal. Each time I check my blood sugar and find it's normal, there's another reason to smile.

With a total transformation in the thought process, there *is not* any "pain" involved with achieving your goal. There might be occasional setbacks – like a plateau – but if you look at them from the right perspective, then a setback is still a pleasurable thing. Maybe your body just needs some time to adjust to the changes you're putting it through. *If you choose to perceive something as painful, then for you it will be painful.*

I choose pleasure.

June 29

A strange thing happened to me in the bathroom today at work, just after I'd finished peeing. When I buckled my pants and was threading the end of the belt through the loops, something just didn't feel right. I lifted my shirt, looked in the mirror, and found that my belt was one notch tighter. And it was perfectly comfortable.

Often, when people want something, they think of it in terms of what they don't want. For example, think about the things people say when they want to quit smoking:

"I don't want to get lung cancer."

"I don't want to spend so much money on cigarettes."

Do you see? They refer to what they *don't* want, not what they want. Perhaps this a minor point, but it's key when I want to set goals for myself. One thing I always keep in mind is that my thoughts control my every action. Some of my "old" ways of thinking about losing weight and choosing health were:

"I don't want to die young."

"I don't want to eat so much junk food."

"I don't want to feel embarrassed any more in public when I think people are staring."

"I don't want to breathe hard when I walk up the stairs."

The key distinction is in the way we state these desires for weight loss. Look at these "wants," this time phrased positively:

"I want to live a long healthy life."

"I want to eat food that's healthy and helps my body."

"I want to go out in public and amaze people with the way I look."

"I want to run up the stairs whenever I want, effortlessly."

Do you see the difference? The first set of statements is totally disabling, and the second set as absolutely empowering. Using thoughts such as these can really help when one wants to set health- or weight-related goals. The following questions are designed to help you to wake your creative side and set a powerful goal for transforming yourself:

Why do I want to lose weight or change my health?

What do I want to gain by changing myself?

What will it cost me physically if I don't begin to change *right now?* Emotionally? Financially?

What is one action can I take *right now* that will take me toward my goal?

What can I accomplish by the end of the week that will move me toward my goal? The end of the month? The end of the year?

Specifically, what do I want to accomplish with my weight and my health?

These questions will help you define exactly the goal you want to set, and to spur the commitment in you to accomplish it. When starting out, it is tempting to make generalized statements like, "I want to lose weight." Questions like the above help to refine the goal to something particular, like, "I want to lose X pounds, and I want to do it by Y, because Z."

Take time with the questions and write down several answers to each. Goals are born from a need to solve a problem, and this exercise will put you in a peak problem-solving state. The more time you spend with the questions and your answers, the more concise your goal will be. As your goal becomes more precise, your commitment to accomplishing the goal grows stronger.

June 30

Once you've written down and answered the questions from the last entry, spend some time reflecting on your answers. Distill your thoughts down to a single sentence or paragraph that will become your goal. The goal is not something you want to do; it is something you will do. Here's mine:

"I will lose enough weight to weigh 190 pounds by the end of May 2001, because my health is worth the change, my family is worth the change, and I'm tired of living in a prison of fat! I am absolutely committed to losing this weight while remaining healthy, eating well, and exercising regularly."

Write your goal down and put it somewhere where you'll see it *daily*. For me, this is my bathroom mirror. I reflect on my goal several times a day and continually reinforce my determination by taking some action towards meeting this goal at every opportunity. Every meal is a chance to take action.

Meeting your goal does not require "willpower," at least not in the usual sense. People believe that weight loss is merely "the willpower not to eat." According to the dictionary, willpower means "energetic determination," so rearranging these statements, we get that weight loss means having an "energetic determination not to eat."

Utter garbage.

What's wrong with that statement? It reeks of deprivation! Any sort of eating plan based on deprivation doesn't work, because it enforces the notion that eating is some sort of moral choice, so that you become "good" or "bad" because of what you put in your mouth. Eating should never be a moral issue, nor should it be the basis of your self-worth.

Once your goal is set, written down, and put in a place where you see it regularly, you can begin taking actions towards realizing the goal. The most important action you can take is to live as though the goal has already been accomplished. Eat like you're the person you want to be; work out like that person; act as if you're that person – and you will become that person.

I imagine weighing 190 pounds. My body realizes that I still weigh considerably more, but my brain can be fooled. Thinking and acting like I weigh 190 completely changes the way I'm looking at food and exercise, because I'm no longer looking at things from a "losing weight" frame of mind. Suddenly, I'm looking at it from the perspective of someone who weighs 190 and merely wants to stay at that weight.

Does that make sense?

For me, the choice is no longer, "I'd better not eat that cookie, I'm trying to lose weight." Instead, it has become, "As a fit and healthy person, I'd rather not have the cookie in me." The second has much more power and a much more positive slant. The power of your actions is directly related to the power of your thoughts.

I do realize that I sound like I'm coming from left field sometimes. I believe the things I write here to be true, but I'm not stupid. The first time I notice one of the techniques I use is not working, I'll change it, and try again.

There's an old saying that makes a lot of sense to me, and is the reason I change my techniques as soon as I find something that's not working: "The definition of insanity is doing the same thing over and over again, and expecting a different result." To be successful at achieving any goal, you have to monitor your progress regularly. If what you're doing is not working, *don't keep doing it*. Modify the approach you take, and try again.

July 2000

335 – 319 *pounds*

July 1

I went to get a haircut today, and the man who normally cuts my hair was on vacation until Wednesday. Luckily for me one of his partners was there, and he was able to fit me in. I'm glad this happened, because he imparted some words to me that really struck a chord, and I want to share my thoughts.

As he was putting the oversized cape around my neck, he commented that his neck "used to be bigger" but was now 17 3/4 inches. He brought this up because though the cape he used was tight on me, he didn't have to go get the special-extra-big one like my normal barber always does.

Ah, I thought to myself, *another person to learn from.* I'm a strong believer in finding people who've done what I want to do, then finding out how they achieved their goal.

I asked him if he meant that he'd lost weight. He said yes, and told me his weight loss story in short order. Basically, he lost about 25 pounds by modifying his eating habits and significantly reducing his intake of animal fat. At the end of his story, he said, "I'm glad I finally woke up and realized how much my eating habits were ruling my life."

Without warning, a big light bulb went on over my head and I remembered an old saying that I picked up somewhere through the years: "Man is born to rule or be ruled."

What a true statement that is! Though I don't know the source of the statement, I suspect that it may have been some great ruler who made it as a testament to his ability to lead people. I don't know. Think about the statement in a purely personal sense. People are often ruled by their behaviors and emotions. I know I was, even though I didn't admit it at the time.

Eating controlled my life. If I was happy and wanted to celebrate, we ordered out. Big. For example, anytime we ordered from the local steak delivery place, I'd generally order (just for myself) two 9-oz beef tip dinners or two rib-eye sandwiches and a baked potato.

If I was stressed for some reason, guess what? A Big Mac, two fish sandwiches, a large order of fries, and an apple pie sure made me feel better. Or, if I was in a pizza mood, a 12- or 16-inch pizza sure took care of me. Yes, the whole pizza.

On the very rare occasions that I was unhappy, I found that a trip to Taco Bell (a steak Gordita supreme, two soft tacos supreme, two bean burritos with sour cream, and a chili-cheese burrito) perked me right back up. If I was feeling like Chinese, nothing said happiness like a quart of General Tso's chicken, a pint of fried rice, two egg rolls, and half of a large order of roast duck.

Does this sound like a man in control?

While I was eating one meal, I'd think about the next. One of the things I've learned since I reached my threshold is that I control my behaviors – they do *not* control me. Not any more. Food is no longer the center of my life, because I'm in charge now, and I'm not planning on abdicating my throne any time soon.

July 2

Everything we do asks an inherent question, from "What color pants will I wear today?" to "Should I read this book in the bedroom or in the den?" The questions we ask ourselves can really govern how we live our lives.

But the most insidious questions start with the phrase "what if," and they can be killers. I believe these kinds of questions are designed to help us sabotage some sort of behavior we fear, if we use them improperly. We've all asked ourselves these kinds of questions, and the questions aren't necessarily always bad in and of themselves. They don't become issues until we allow them to become our focus. In reality, the questions can actually help us prepare for potential challenges down the road. The best way I've found to deal with them when they come up is to immediately answer the question with a positive and reaffirming statement.

What if I fail?

I won't fail because I'm committed to making this happen. If I find that what I'm doing is not working, rather than quit, I will simply change the approach I'm taking and try again. All I have to do is be conscious of the results I'm getting, and adjust accordingly.

What makes me think I can do it this time, since all the other tries haven't worked?

I understand that the times I've tried to lose weight in the past have no bearing at all on what I'm doing this time. My past efforts do not dictate my future results.

What if I haven't lost any weight this week?

I realize that there will be weeks when my body is adjusting to a new way of life and that a weight loss of this magnitude will take some time. If I feel that what I'm doing is not working, I'll take the actions described in the answer to "What if I fail?"

Why do I have to exercise every day?

Part of being fit and healthy involves being more active and moving my body around regularly. The exercise helps every part of me – spirit, mind, and body – and is something I *choose* to do, not something I *have* to do.

July 3

Yesterday I focused on some of the negative questions we ask ourselves. I'd like to turn that around today and look at some of the ways I use positive questions to influence my direction.

One thing I firmly believe is that the human brain is one of the world's greatest creations, and as such, my brain can give me an answer to any question I ask it. Remember, though, your brain will give you an answer to any question you ask, so stick to positive questions.

For example, suppose I ask my brain a question like "Why am I such a big fat pig?" My brain is going to do its *best* look for an answer to this. Examine the question closely, however. See the presupposition there? My question is already assuming that I really *am* a "big fat pig!" Questions like these beg for abusive answers. My brain, hearing this question, almost immediately shouts back: "Because you shovel food in your face every time you get near the kitchen!"

Ouch.

Instead of berating myself with my questions, I try to make the questions I ask geared more towards finding an honest answer:

How can I safely and reasonably become a healthy and fit person?

Ah, a completely different mindset now. My brain can rattle off pages and pages of answers to that question, all of them good.

How can I become fit and healthy, and make it fun at the same time?

My brain went to town on that question, and as a result I'm experiencing more joy in my life than I can remember. My wife can vouch for that. I cannot tell these days if I get more energy from exercising and eating well or from all the mind candy I give myself. All I can say for sure is that I'm practically bouncing off the walls, whereas before May 28 I was taking naps almost every single day (sitting at a desk all day tired me out), and now I don't. I've even managed to make riding my stationary bike downright enjoyable, a small miracle.

How can I eat healthy foods after a lifetime of eating unhealthy foods?

This is another example of a question that begs for good answers. I've written already about some of the techniques I use, most notably the visualization of my future self (June 30) and questions for setting a goal (June 29), so I'm not going to cover them again here.

How about I ask myself this question again, but even *more* positively?

How can I eat healthy foods after a lifetime of eating unhealthy foods, and make it fun at the same time?

Try it. You'll be amazed at what your brain will tell you. Ask the questions with the full expectation that you'll get a good answer back. You might get a whole list of answers right away, or they may come to you gradually over a day or two. You've done this before, whether you recognized it or not. Have you ever discovered the solution to a challenge while sitting on the toilet, taking a shower, or even in a dream? I have. This is just your brain giving you the answer to a question you asked it. You may have forgotten you asked, but your brain didn't.

July 4

One emotion that I allowed to rule me for a good part of my fat life was fear. A lot of people are afraid when they confront a massive life-change, and that's perfectly understandable. Humans have a tendency to fear the unknown, and for me, life as a fit, healthy man was very unknown. I believe that the "fear" was a response to the size of my task – and understanding that there was an entire set of core beliefs that I needed to change.

One of the most limiting beliefs I had was the belief that I would fail this time because I had failed before. Most people trying to accomplish a goal (eating right, losing weight, getting healthy, wealthy, whatever) suffer from this same fear if they've ever tried and failed before. This fear is particularly debilitating, because it can make you stop trying before you've even started.

Luckily, dealing with this fear is not terribly difficult. Realize that no matter what you've done or tried in the past to reach your goal in no way affects the future. That's some serious power. You can start each day fresh and new. Stop thinking about how you've failed in the past, even if it happened just yesterday! I cannot stress this enough: don't dwell on the past, because you cannot change it. You can only live for the present and for the future.

Another fear we deal with is the fear of success. Standing on the 371-pound side of a 183-pound weight loss is a daunting thing. Some interesting questions arise:

What happens if I lose all this weight and just gain it right back?

Will I still be the same person when this is over?

What if I lose the weight and I still have problems with my diabetes?

All of these questions lead to one place only: the belief that success will lead to some kind of new pain, be it mental or physical. Deal with this fear by reaffirming the huge amount of pleasure that waits at the end of the road. Here are a few pleasure items that help me:

- *When I reach my goal, I'll have more energy in my life than I've ever had before.*
- *I will be able to shop in a normal clothing store, instead of at "King Size Male."*
- *My health will be increased a hundred-fold.*

- *I can go to the mall without constantly plucking at the front of my shirt and worrying about people staring at me.*
- *I can climb a ladder without worrying about its maximum load.*
- *I can dance with my wife.*

Looking at this list, I just realized that my statements went from "I will" to "I can" right in the middle. This was purely unconscious on my part, and I didn't notice it till I was finished making the list. This is exactly the sort of thing I mean when I talk about living as though you'd already accomplished your goals.

What happens when I start writing down, or at the very least listing in my head, the pleasurable things about changing my lifestyle, I find that they greatly outnumber the few negative thoughts I was having. With such sheer volume and power, it's easy to determine valid answers to the fear questions from above, and thereby break the hold the fear has on me.

What happens if I lose all this weight and just gain it right back?

As someone who is totally committed to a lifetime of health, there is no chance that this can happen. I know that if I start to regain any weight, I will immediately experience significant emotional pain. Since my brain is already wired to avoid pain, it will lead me to get right back to the weight I've chosen for myself.

Will I still be the same person when this is over?

Of course I will! I'll just be happier, more energetic, and have even more passion for life than I do now!

What if I lose the weight and I still have problems with my diabetes?

My doctor told me that I could completely control my diabetes with my diet, and I believe that. No matter what happens with my diabetes when I lose this weight, it cannot be nearly as bad as it is now.

Allow yourself to be fear-free, and your world will open up.

July 7

One of the most powerful ways to overcome a fear is to simply confront it, and realize that you are bigger than it will ever be. Be aware that most of your fears are not fears of something tangible; they are only fears of possibility.

I'd like to touch back on what I believe is the biggest fear most people have: the fear of failure. This is the most paralyzing fear there is because it makes you stop before you ever try. The fear of failure drains your energy and can bring about a life that is not really about living at all. In life, according to an old saying, there are three kinds of people – those who make things happen, those who watch things happen, and those who say, "What happened?"

Which kind of person do you choose to be?

To confront the fear of failure and destroy it, it's important to overcome the mindset that failing is a bad thing. Thomas Edison, while trying to invent the light bulb, had over 10,000 failures before he got it right. A reporter asked him how he felt about so many failures, and his response was, "I have not failed, I have just found 10,000 ways that don't work."

Let's make it a little more personal. When you were a child, how many times did you try to learn to ride a bike before you gave up? One time? Five times? Since most people know how to ride a bike, my guess is that you didn't give up. When you were fifteen or sixteen, and you found out that you had to turn the wheel, work the clutch, move the gearshift, and watch the road on all four sides at the same time, did you decide to ride your bike instead?

I can still remember sitting in the church parking lot with my father in his VW Super Beetle as he explained the whole idea of the clutch to me. I was excited at the prospect of becoming even closer to being grown up, and didn't pay a lot of attention. I got the basic idea that I needed to put the clutch in and let it out every time I needed to change gears.

Want to guess what happened the first time I actually tried using the clutch? I stalled the car. That also happened the second, third, fourth, and even the fifth time. Finally I thought to myself, *maybe you should pay more attention to this man beside you*. He explained once again that I should release the clutch slowly, rather than just popping it out.

I tried again, slowly this time, and the car nudged forward. Elated, I popped the clutch the rest of the way out, and promptly stalled out again.

It took time, but I did it, and I'm still driving to this day. The difference now is that the whole process is so ingrained that I do it automatically.

When I achieve the results I want with regards to my health, they too will become automatic after a while.

For those of you with children, how many times did you watch them fall down while learning to walk, before you gave up on them and bought them a wheelchair?

Personally, I don't care for the word "fail." To fail means to be unsuccessful, and the only people who are unsuccessful are the people who never try. Instead of framing my actions in emotional words like "succeed" and "fail," I use the word "results." Think about it. Any time you do something, you get results. These results might be the results you wanted, or they might not.

When I decided to transform from my old life to my new life, I knew there were some specific results I wanted. They included lowering my blood sugar to the point where I no longer required medicine, and to where I possessed an abundance of energy and a new sense of well being about my body, and finally, to achieve significant weight loss.

I've taken some pretty massive actions to make changes. Right now I'm watching my results, and so far I'm happy with them. The key to "success" is to continually monitor your results. If I ever get results I don't want, I will simply reevaluate the whole situation, and what I'm doing. Once I have reevaluated, I will again take a different action and watch my results. This process will go on and on, refining itself, until I'm exactly where I want to be.

Persist, and you can never fail.

July 10

I've been giving a lot of thought recently to the things I say, because one of my strongest beliefs is that words have power. What I say with regards to food and eating can directly impact changes I'm making in my life, and it's time for a vocabulary change.

For example, consider the phrase "I'm starving," and all its variants. These include "I could eat a horse," "I'm dying of starvation," "I'll faint if I don't eat soon," and a plethora of related terms. Look at that for a minute. Am I really going to starve if I don't put something in my mouth immediately? No. These statements are patently false, and they serve to either cause or justify overeating.

Consider: if you constantly tell your brain that you're starving, what kind of message are you sending it? While the statement may not be consciously believed, it sends an incorrect message to your subconscious. Because the subconscious mind cannot differentiate between fact and fiction, sending it messages like that merely serve to cause it confusion.

Any time I catch myself saying or thinking something like this now, I try to stop it immediately, and even have an internal conversation with myself.

"Self," I say in my head, to avoid strange looks, "are you *really* starving?"

Begrudgingly, my self answers, "No."

"Are you merely hungry? Is that all? Am I in any danger of immediate demise?"

Again the response is in the negative.

"In that case, would you shut up? I know I'm hungry without you trying to cloud the issue!"

And, with a sniff of disdain, my self shuts right up.

Another word I refuse to use is the word "diet." I'm not referring to the noun form of the word, because that's just the foods we eat. The form of the word I abhor is the more insidious form, the verb. The action word that means you should eat and drink sparingly or according to prescribed rules. This word is all about deprivation, and my complete and total belief on deprivation is that we tend to crave anything we feel that we cannot have. Imagine someone telling you that you can never have any more Coke, or Oreos, or steak, or something else you may really like.

Don't get me wrong, I know I don't *need* to eat those things, but I *can* if I choose to. See? It's all about choices. I can have a bag of Oreos, but I choose not to at this time. You may think it's all a matter of semantics (and you may be right), but the subtle changes in your mind add up to one big change in your body.

July 13

I'd like to discuss a few specific words I use that need changing. The first such word is "lose" in its various forms – lose, losing, lost – in regards to one's weight. There are several definitions for this word in the dictionary, including:

"To suffer deprivation of: part with especially in an unforeseen or accidental manner"

"To undergo deprivation of something of value"

"To suffer loss from"

"To undergo defeat"

Still feel like "losing" a little weight?

I say no to this word, "lose," unequivocally. I know I sometimes sound a little odd, but as of today, I'm 46 days into my decision to make a change, and I weigh 43 pounds less. I haven't starved, and I certainly haven't deprived myself. The only suffering I go through is the pins and needles in my butt that I get when it goes numb on the stationary bike.

There's no chance of my weight winning any sort of victory over me, because I'm not fighting it. There's no battle to be won here. I've made a decision to live, act, exercise, and eat like a 190-pound man, and I truly believe that's all it takes. I'm not "losing" weight, I'm shedding pounds of fat that my body no longer needs or wants. And for the record, unlike others shedding weight, I don't consider myself a "loser."

I'm a winner.

July 14

One of the words I find myself using regularly is "change," which I've started using describing what I've done in my life. Think of "change" as the alternative to things like "I'm trying to lose weight" or "I'm losing weight" or even "I'm on a diet." A glance at the dictionary under the heading "change" yields the following:

"To make a shift from one to another"

"To become different"

"To undergo transformation"

"To shift to a new purpose"

All of these are incredibly positive, because they indicate I'm a whole new person. Combining some of them, I see "to shift from an old purpose to a new purpose," which is exactly what I've done.

Once upon a time, food was a primary source of pleasure to me. The transformation I've undergone and continue to undergo allows me to see food for what it really is: fuel for my body. Don't get me wrong, I still believe I can get pleasure from what I eat, but the focus has changed. I'm the one in charge now.

July 15

A word of advice: If, by chance, you find yourself in the deep south of the United States in the middle of July, and you furthermore happen to find yourself outside on a beautiful clear sunny day when the temperature is 98 degrees Fahrenheit, and you decide to stay outside on said day from noon until 1:30 pm in the direct light of the sun, working on cleaning your pool and installing a fountain, make sure you don't leave 90% of your body uncovered.

The fountain does look good, though.

July 16

When I got home from grocery shopping yesterday morning, I loaded myself up with as much as I could possibly carry and came inside, where I immediately saw my new scales. These scales are digital medical scales that I ordered online, and they weigh correctly all the way up to 500 pounds, unlike most scales, which only go to 300 or 350.

I jumped on the scales holding all this food, and checked the scales. 367. Holding all that food, I still weighed four pounds less than when I started. I cannot see how I ever made it up the stairs when I weighed 371, because at 367 (carrying the groceries) I thought I was going to collapse in a heap and tumble back down to the bottom. I suppose having the weight spread all over my body made it more tolerable than having it all suspended at the ends of my arms, but either way it was a rough trip upstairs, and my arms thanked me profusely when I put the groceries down on the counter in the kitchen.

July 17

I think I've gotten my visualization of the new me down pat. I'm thinking so differently now that I've managed to forget to eat breakfast until around 10:00 am both yesterday and today.

Will the miracles never cease?

❧

Sabotage. Isn't that an ugly word? It means "deliberate subversion," and I see and speak with people daily who do it to themselves with regards to their weight. It's frightening, because people seem to be doing so well at achieving their goals, then suddenly it's all for naught. I'm not talking about shedding three pounds and then eating fast food for a few days and gaining it all back. No, these are people who achieve wonderful things over the course of several months, getting rid of 30, 40, 50, or more pounds. Suddenly, though, almost overnight it seems they just stop and in almost no time they've gained back everything they'd shed.

So they start again.

Seeing this all around me, I wonder what it is that makes people do this. More importantly, will I do it in the near future? What can happen to a person to make them just give up and revert back to their old ways? I have done it before; how can I prevent it from happening again?

One of the biggest reasons we slide back into our old ways is that we don't initially associate enough pain with changing. I realize some people may not care for my use of the word "pain," here, so think of it as "discomfort," if you'd rather. Pain/pleasure, comfort/discomfort, the dichotomy is the same. We tend to move towards one and away from the other.

We get caught up in the heat of the moment and feel a little pain with the thought of not getting rid of excess weight, and desire to make a change. This works for a while, but inevitably, the combination of the short term pain of changing and the pleasure of eating those wickedly decadent foods comes back, and we slide right back into our original state – or worse, we gain *more* weight back. Talk about pain!

The key is that the pain associated with *not* changing has to be significant. It has to be massive pain, because that's the only real pain strong enough to elicit a complete changing of your life. For me, this pain was seeing someone have to have his leg removed because he didn't take care of himself. He and I had a lot in common, we did, in that we both had been diagnosed with diabetes but hadn't been taking care of ourselves. Lucky for me I got to see his example, and not become one myself.

I wish, truly, that there were some magical words I could say or something I could do to show everyone I meet how to find their pain, but it's a personal process. You have to look inside yourself, and see what it is that would give you the desire, the motivation, to change your life in a flash. It's a transformation, really, and it's instant when you find it. It's not a gradual thing.

Perhaps you'll feel your clothes getting tighter and realize you don't want to spend the rest of your life buying bigger and bigger outfits. Maybe you're tired of wheezing when you walk up a single flight of stairs. It could be that you want to be able to play with your kids for hours on end, rather than just watching them play from the comfort of a chair on the porch.

If you look for it, you'll find it.

July 19

Lying in bed last night, waiting for Robyn to finish brushing her teeth, my muse tossed a word into my head that describes my situation exactly: liberate, in its various forms. One definition of "liberate" is "to release from combination." If you think of my fat and my body as being in combination, I'm "liberating" the fat from my body. I like that! It's much prettier than "losing weight," "getting rid of weight," or "shedding weight."

A second definition of the word "liberate" means "to set free." We humans are unique in that we create situations and problems for ourselves where we manage to be both the prisoner and the jailer. Though I've been locked in this prison for eighteen years, I've only been there because I never seriously tried to open the door.

July 20

When I tell people about the amount of fat I've liberated, they get pretty excited and want to know my "secret." Specifically, they want to know what diet I'm on. Generally, I respond with, "I'm not on a diet; I eat whatever I want to," which is perhaps a little misleading. I eat whatever I choose, the key being the word "choose." I know that I can *have* a Snickers bar, or some Little Debbie, but I *choose* not to.

By choosing mostly foods that are healthful, I'm well on the way to becoming the man I see in my head. I choose well because the thought of eating unhealthy foods causes me pain, and I feel incredible pleasure from eating things I know are helping my body. Would it be possible to eat mostly unhealthy foods and still liberate the fat from my body? Sure, but that wouldn't be in the best interests of my health. I'm in this for the long haul.

Also key in this quest for health is exercise. Exercise: it burns calories, it works out the heart, it helps breathing, it builds stamina, and it increases my metabolism. Up until May 28, I considered exercise to be massive pain, and chose instead to sit on my butt most of the time. After I made my necessary mental changes, exercise became pleasurable for me.

July 21

If I speak in the tongues of men and of angels, but have not love, I am only a resounding gong or a clanging cymbal. If I have the gift of prophecy and can fathom all mysteries and all knowledge, and if I have a faith that can move mountains, but have not love, I am nothing. If I give all I possess to the poor and surrender my body to the flames, but have not love, I gain nothing.

Love is patient, love is kind. It does not envy, it does not boast, it is not proud. It is not rude, it is not self-seeking, it is not easily angered, it keeps no record of wrongs. Love does not delight in evil but rejoices with the truth. It always protects, always trusts, always hopes, always perseveres.

Love never fails. But where there are prophecies, they will cease; where there are tongues, they will be stilled; where there is knowledge, it will pass away. For we know in part and we prophesy in part, but when perfection comes, the imperfect disappears. When I was a child, I talked like a child, I thought like a child, I reasoned like a child. When I became a man, I put childish ways behind me. Now we see but a poor reflection as in a mirror; then we shall see face to face. Now I know in part; then I shall know fully, even as I am fully known.

And now these three remain: faith, hope, and love. But the greatest of these is love. – I Corinthians 13 (NIV)

One thing I've learned since I decided to transform myself is that in order to love other people effectively, you must love yourself first. I spent a good deal of my life not loving myself. When I looked in the mirror I saw a fat, ugly, disgusting person that no one could ever love. As I got fatter and fatter, I stopped going out into public, because I believed people were staring at me due to my size. Somewhere inside, I was still the little chubby kid that got picked last because he was fat.

And then I met my wife, who showed me I was lovable.

That helped me a lot, and still helps me to this day, but after she moved here to be with me, I still kept getting fatter and fatter, because I hadn't truly let go of the self-hatred. From the time she moved here in August 1996 until May of this year, I blossomed up an additional 40 pounds or so from my already superfat 330 pounds.

I became a blob that could walk until I realized that I'd be nothing as a person as long as I didn't love myself. I'm not talking about narcissism, I'm talking about self-love: the unconditional acceptance of myself.

Self-love encourages people to love us, and allows us to accept their love. Without self-love, we too easily reject the love of others because we don't recognize it.

Self-love also feels pretty damn good. It's a definite pleasure, and allows us to understand ourselves at a deeper level, because we're not hiding anything from ourselves any more.

So, you're thinking right now, if you're not already a lover of self, *that sounds good, Fred, but how can I start to love myself?*

Good question. The easiest way I've found to increase self love is to simply tell yourself: "I love myself."

I'm all for simple answers.

It might sound hokey and laughable, but it works. I'm not talking about saying it on occasion; I'm talking about saying it 50 to 100 times a day. In just a few days, you'll notice a difference. Try and prove me wrong!

Try this, too: see yourself being kind to yourself, and loving yourself, and before you know it, you're there. Act as if you already love yourself. Does this sound familiar yet?

Make an effort to be forgiving towards both yourself and other people.

Get rid of shame – if you make a mistake, learn from it and don't wallow in it. Shame does nothing more than make you feel that there's something innately wrong and undeserving within you. If you're feeling shame, it's impossible to love yourself or to allow yourself to be loved.

July 22

The only reality we know is that which we perceive. Our outlook on life is formed by our past experiences, and everything going into our brains as input is filtered through that outlook. The way we react to any given situation is based on our perception of that situation. Change your perceptions, and you change your reality.

Think about it for a second. What is your belief about people in general? Do you believe people are basically kind, helpful, and good, or do you believe they're bad, out to get you, or even evil? Take some time to reflect on how you feel about others. My guess is, if you look back into your past, you can find specific examples to support your belief.

A belief is nothing more than a sense of certainty that an idea is true. It forms the filter that creates reality for each of us. I used to believe that because I was so fat, I was worthless as a person and unlovable. Furthermore, I believed the stereotype that fat people are lazy, which in turn made me never want to get off my butt and do anything.

I believe that we all are the masters of our own destiny, and that our beliefs and perceptions shape that destiny. What sort of destiny do you think I had while I believed I was worthless, lazy, and unlovable? Was I just "getting by" or was I designing a life that would be memorable?

There are two words that can immediately start to transform our perceptions, and therefore our reality. These words are "I am," and they carry a power like the world has never known.

I am lovable. I am a valuable human being. I am hardworking.

Say them once, and you grin because you feel like an idiot. Say them ten times, and you start to wonder if you're going slightly batty. Say them one hundred times, and you start to believe them. Say them one thousand times, and they become your reality. I don't think there's any small significance to the fact that in the Bible, God referred to Himself as "I am." I've said it before, and I'll say it again: your subconscious mind believes everything you tell it, and will create any reality for you that you want.

I am a fit man who weighs 190 pounds and is wonderfully healthy.

I visited my doctor on Thursday for some blood work. My blood sugar was 89, less than two hours after eating lunch. My doctor believes that coming off the diabetes medication within the next year won't be an issue, because for all intents and purposes, I won't be a diabetic any more.

With faith, all things are possible.

July 24

My week was made today by a customer who chased me down as I was leaving his site. He followed me down the hall calling for me to wait, and we exchanged greetings. Right after, he proclaimed, "What have you done to *lose so much weight?*"

Like I said, it made my week.

❧

As a software engineer, I tend to see many things in life in computer terms. I think of my brain as a giant, powerful computer which I can program myself, or which I can allow those around me to program.

Instead of a monitor, a keyboard, an Internet connection, a microphone, and a mouse, I've got my senses: hearing, seeing, feeling, tasting, and smelling. These senses give my brain the same sorts of inputs that computer peripherals give to a CPU. Everything I've ever learned or done is stored in my RAM (short term memory) or on my hard drive (long term memory).

The backbone of this wonderful computer is its central processing unit, the subconscious mind. The subconscious is a phenomenal multitasking system, running your entire body at once. It uses the autonomic nervous system to control your involuntary actions like breathing, heartbeat, and digestion. It also handles all of the input from your five senses simultaneously, and processes all the thoughts your conscious mind is feeding it.

Imagine if you had to control via your conscious mind all the different things your subconscious mind does. Life would suddenly change from being a rich experience into merely trying to survive. Scientists estimate that of the entity we call our "mind" the subconscious portion is about 90%-95% and the conscious mind is only about 5%-10%, because that's all that's needed to deal with the "here and now."

Have you ever had a time when you were desperately trying to think of something, perhaps the title of a song or book, and you couldn't. You knew it, it was on the tip of your tongue, but you couldn't get it out so you gave up and forgot about it. Then, sometime later when you were sitting around doing nothing, you got a funny look on your face, almost confused, and shouted out the answer to whatever you were looking for earlier, causing everyone around you to jump and stare suspiciously at you. Even funnier, if any of the same people who were there when you were trying to get that answer are still around, chances are they immediately said, "Oh yeah!"

I like to imagine that there's a little man living in my head – a personification of my subconscious, if you will. He's sitting at a desk behind a window, looking out at my conscious mind. When I need something, the request sails through the window and lands on his desk.

He jumps up, and begins scanning through every experience I've ever had, looking for the answer to this request. This may take some time, because he's got a lot of memory to search. Usually, though, he's able to get the answer back out pretty quickly.

In cases like the scenario above, where you're trying your darnedest to remember something, I believe what happens is something like this:

1) You send the initial request to your little man, and he gets busy.
2) This particular answer happens to be cross-linked, requiring a linear search and therefore using more time.
3) On the conscious side, you get a little impatient with the amount of time he's taking, so you resubmit the question.
4) The little man has to stop looking to come back to the desk to see what it is you want, which just serves to delay him.
5) Go back to step 1, until you stop asking the question.

Once you've forgotten about the question, you free him up to finish his search. When he's found what you're looking for, he races back to his desk and *screams* "Forty-two!" or whatever your answer happens to be, causing you to jump and do the same, eliciting the aforementioned looks from your friends.

This little man is very powerful, because he can do anything you want him to. He doesn't have to just sit at his desk all day long, looking up trivia answers for you. You can control him, and make him create for you whatever it is that you desire.

July 25

Like all CPUs, our brain has its own language and runs programs constantly. Everything our subconscious controls, like our heartbeat or digestion, is just one big program. Other things we do subconsciously are also programs, like walking, driving, and eating.

We also run emotional programs daily, totally unconsciously. Many of the "problems" we have are really just simple programs that we've written to our mental hard drives and run on a regular basis. Depression, overeating, anger, unhappiness, and worry are all programs. For example there are people who, any time a challenge arises, hang their heads, slump their shoulders, and proclaim, "I'm so unhappy!"

I'm no psychologist, but here's what I think may have happened. One day, long ago, one of these people was overwhelmed by some situation, and became unhappy. Someone, perhaps a parent, patted them on the back and said something like, "It's okay, things will work out," which gave that person a good feeling. Repeating this a few times ingrained it as a program. The source code (language that makes up a program) for his program might look like this (this is called pseudo-code in my line of work; it's English words that explain what code does. Everything after a // in a line is just a comment):

```
program I_am_unhappy;
begin
    call Overwhelmed(work); // This is another program!
    call Speak("I am unhappy!"); // Still another!
    if GetResponse("It's OK") then exit // Stop the program
    else repeat I_am_unhappy;
end;
```

Do you see what happens? The person looks for a particular response, and if he doesn't get it, he just cycles the program endlessly and remains unhappy.

Before I changed my life, I ran several of my own mental programs with regards to eating. For example, if I watch TV, it's generally at night. My program with regards to TV-watching was basically "if the TV is on and it's night time, I need to eat something while I watch." Not terribly conducive to the healthy lifestyle, is it?

Here's another: "if I call my Boredom program, and it returns a value of True, then I need to go look in the kitchen for some food." This is a particularly heinous program, because it's *far* too easy to get your Boredom program to return a True to you. Simple, and deadly.

The trick in reprogramming your mind is fairly simple, but what it requires first is that you recognize that you are, in fact, running a program, when it is happening. For this, you have to actually pay a little attention to what you are doing, and merely watch for them. They're really not all that hard to find.

July 27

When programming, sometimes you have errors in your code (we call these "bugs") that need fixing. To find and fix these errors, software engineers use a tool called a debugger and put breakpoints in the faulty code to test certain things at that point in the code's execution. A breakpoint is nothing more than an interruption in the code that a designer uses to find bugs or to modify the code's behavior at runtime.

To successfully reprogram or delete a program that's not running the way we desire, we breakpoint the program while it's running. Break it enough times and it's forever gone, which gives you a fresh slate on which to start rewriting.

I enjoy testing my theories not only on myself, but on those around me too. Earlier, I talked about people who run an "I'm so unhappy" program. If you should encounter one of these people, instead of giving them the feedback they want, take the opportunity to put a breakpoint in their program. The conversation might look something like this:

Person: "I'm so unhappy!"

You: "Congratulations! How'd you manage to do it?" (Right here is the breakpoint. They won't know what hit them.)

Person: "What?"

You: "It takes a lot of effort, being that unhappy. I'm proud of you for doing something so hard!" (Big smile to them here)

Person, looking confused: "Pardon?"

You, smiling all the time: "Well, you've got to hang your head, and look down, and get your shoulders all slumped over, and make yourself feel bad, and that's a hell of a lot of work. I don't think I could do it."

Person walks away, smiling.

See how that worked? It breaks their program, and snaps them right out of their unhappy state. Doing this once won't elicit a permanent change, but continually breaking their pattern will have a definite effect – as long as other people aren't reinforcing their program.

Breaking a program doesn't always have to be outrageous and comical, like that one, but outrageousness can break the really firmly entrenched ones. The real key is to be able to recognize the program, so that you can breakpoint it. Once you've recognized it, and find yourself running it, do something loud or obnoxious that will instantly stop the program. Then, all you have to do is choose a different way to run the program, or to remove it altogether.

Above all, have fun while you do it. Life's too short not to.

July 28

In the last twenty-four hours, on two separate occasions, people have told me they don't like themselves very much these days, and asked for advice on how to deal with that. So, as my thought for the day, I offer this:

Get a piece of paper and a pen, and sit down in a quiet place. Write down a list of at least 25 things you like about yourself. Take the time to think your items through, and list (in your head) reasons to back up those items. Meditate on the items, and remember that you're worth loving.

July 29

As persons, we are 100% responsible for our beliefs, our thoughts, and our actions. All too often overweight people want to look somewhere else for blame for their size:

- *"I have a gland problem."*
- *"I have big bones."*
- *"My parents didn't love me."*
- *"I was beaten as a child."*
- *"I was raped."*
- *"I was sexually abused."*
- *"I'm clinically depressed."*

I'm not trying to make light of anyone's past, and believe me I think all forms of abuse are horrible. In no way is it my intention to minimize the experiences of someone's life. But regardless of our past, however, there's absolutely no reason why it needs to be allowed to control either the present or the future. It's over. Period. If you continue to let your past control you, you remain a victim, and life as a victim is no sort of fulfilling life at all. Release it, and move forward. Grow.

Responsibility brings with it a wonderful sense of power. This power gives you the ability to control your own destiny. You cannot always control what happens to you, but you can control how you choose to respond to it. Your future is only what you choose for it to be.

July 31

When you come to the realization that you are responsible for your life and your destiny, you're suddenly imbued with a wonderful power – the power of choice. A responsible person is no longer a victim because he knows he has the ability to choose his responses. A responsible person understands that he got to be almost 200 pounds over his ideal weight because of the choices he made about what, when, and how much to eat over the course of his life. He knows that at any instant in time, he can choose to make different, more healthy and nutritious, choices. A responsible person can respond to cruelty in others with cruelty and hate, or he can choose to respond with forgiveness and love.

A responsible person can give up in the face of adversity, or he can choose to prevail. W. Mitchell is a well-known motivational speaker. He's also an author, a former mayor, was responsible for the passage of the Americans with Disabilities Act, and is a millionaire many times over.

He did this all after surviving not only a motorcycle wreck that gave him third-degree burns over 70% of his body, but also a plane crash that paralyzed him from the waist down.

A responsible person can look at the weight liberation process as "hard," "difficult," "a battle," or "a war," or he can choose to view it as a simple change of habits. It's only as difficult as you choose to believe.

Every single thing that happens in your life gives you a choice, and every choice you make has a specific outcome that will affect you. As the character says at the end of *Indiana Jones and the Last Crusade*, you can choose wisely or you can choose poorly.

How will you choose?

August 2000

319 – 300 *pounds*

August 2

When a pilot flies an airplane from one city to another, his path is never a straight line. He has to constantly monitor his progress during the flight, because several things present themselves as obstacles during his journey. Wind can cause a gradual drift off the plotted course, and turbulent winds can cause very dramatic shifts in a plane's direction. Other planes, airports, and natural landscape items such as mountains must be avoided. A pilot has to contend with the rotation of the Earth during a flight, lest he completely miss his destination.

If a pilot is not continually vigilant, and entirely focused on where he wants to go, he'll either end up the wrong city, or as a flaming piece of debris in a field somewhere. Neither of these is conducive to his happiness, the happiness of the airline, or the happiness of the passengers.

Much in the same way, a person who has made a decision to regain lost health or to shed excess fat must constantly monitor his progress. The temptations surrounding him are like the wind, sometimes gently pushing him adrift, sometimes knocking him completely off the path with their siren call. Friends and loved ones who aren't supportive of him are obstacles in his path to be avoided, lest he crash and burn. A failure to continually watch his actions will allow him to fall right back into his old habits, and will lead to a final state that is worse than his original one.

Most people fail in their quest to change their lifestyle because they lack constant focus. Stay focused, and you'll achieve any goal you set for yourself. Lose your focus, and never succeed.

August 4

Are you a labeler? Lots of people are, it seems, constantly giving themselves labels and thus excuses for their behavior.

- *I couldn't help eating that whole cake, my psychiatrist says I'm depressed.*
- *I'm as sick as a dog, so I cannot work out.*
- *I'm in a bad mood; eating a bag of cookies will help.*
- *I cannot exercise because I'm too tired.*

The list can go on without end. I am not saying these aren't valid problems. However, they are not valid excuses for certain behaviors. All labeling yourself does is reinforce some particular belief you may have. I won't go so far as to say that I think changing your label will change you, but I certainly think it helps you on your way to wholeness. That's the best reason for why I refuse to define myself as a diabetic.

Are you letting your labels define who you are as a person?

August 6

Thoughts influence speech. These words, in turn, direct and enforce our beliefs, which cause us to take specific actions, and produce the results we see. Our results have an influence on our thoughts, and start the whole process over, again and again. I think of this whole process as the cycle of change, and it can be envisioned as a big circle.

One good thing to note in this cycle is that it can be interrupted at any point to create a new cycle. For example, by simply changing the words you use, whether you believe them or not, you can create a new cycle where the words actually become true and you do believe them. The important thing to realize is that the further into the circle you break, the worse your chances are for changing the cycle completely. For the maximum change in a cycle, start with changing your thoughts.

Scientists estimate that the average person has about 60,000 unique thoughts per day. This is a phenomenal number. It's about one per second, if you don't count sleeping time. There's a kicker to this, though. Scientists also estimate that 95% of those thoughts are the *same* thoughts that person had yesterday. We humans are amazingly habitual creatures, and it's no wonder so many people fail when they start a new weight-shedding program. By changing their eating habits, they're breaking into the circle above at the "actions" point, which is too late in the cycle to cause lasting change.

When you break into the circle at the "actions" point, you'll see some initial limited results, nowhere nearly as fast as you want, because you're still thinking, speaking, and believing like a fat person. You get limited results from your diet, and you move the cycle just a tiny bit, but habit brings it right back where it was before. I've seen it happen far too many times. You're not going to the results you want until you first change your underlying thoughts about yourself.

Become, in your head, the person you want to be. When I look in the mirror, I don't see a 300+ pound morbidly obese diabetic man. Instead, I see a 190-pound fit man with no health problems, who is, in fact, the definition of health. I see this and I believe it with all my heart. When I'm in bed at night I think about how nice it is to be so healthy. When I wake up in the morning I stretch and marvel over how good it feels to be in such good shape – even if I'm sore. When it's time to eat I think about eating healthy choices for my new 190-pound body.

If you want to make a lasting change in yourself, start with changing your thoughts first. You cannot always control some of your thoughts, but you can certainly suppress the ones you don't want when they bubble up. Lest you think I'm completely full of hogwash, look at what some of the world's most well known thinkers have to say about the power of thought.

"We are what we think. All that we are arises with our thoughts. With our thoughts, we make our world." – Buddha

"A man's what he thinks about all day long" – Ralph Waldo Emerson

"Why should we think upon things that are lovely? Because thinking determines life. It is a common habit to blame life upon the environment. Environment modifies life but does not govern life. The soul is stronger than its surroundings." – William James

"As [a man] thinks in his heart, so is he" – Proverbs 23:7 (NKJV)

August 7

I went to the fat man's store today to buy a new belt, because mine is now too large. I also bought a couple of pairs of pants, and brought them home without trying them on. I'm pleased to announce that the 48-inch waist pants I bought today are loose on me. Not so loose that 46's would fit, but loose nonetheless. This means nothing to you unless you understand that I started at a comfortable 54.

❧

In addition to changing our thoughts, changing our words can have a tremendous effect on our results. Think about it for a minute, and let's look at something simple. If someone asks you an innocuous question like, "How's it going?" what sort of answer do you usually give?

"Okay."

"So-so."

"Crappy."

"My life sucks."

What do you think happens if you tell yourself these things over and over again every day? Do you think there's a chance you'll start to believe them? Do you think they'll affect your quality of life? I do. If there's one thing I've learned in this life, it is this: words have an effect. You may not notice the effect instantly, but I guarantee they'll have one.

Take for example, the person who constantly says, "I'm so depressed!" Is it not possible that that person is just reinforcing his thoughts and in turn getting a belief in his head that he is, in fact, a depressed person? What sort of results will that produce on his actions and the results he has in his life?

When I respond to a question like "How's it going?" I use words like "terrific," "wonderful," "superb," "phenomenal," and "exquisite." Do I always feel that good? Maybe not, but you know what happens? As soon I tell someone I feel that way, using one of those words, it starts to make me feel that way just a little.

Now, let's look briefly at some of the words we use when talking about aspects of food:

"I'm starving!"

"I'll die if I don't eat soon!"

"I could eat a horse!"

Can you see where these words can pretty easily lead someone to overeat when sitting down for a meal? What would happen if you simply modified what you said to something along the lines of "I'm a tad hungry," or "I think my body needs a little nourishment?" It sounds hokey, but you'll be surprised how it can change your state of hunger. Our words have power.

August 8

When I was a kid, I read the entire *Little House* series of books. In one of them, Laura asks her Pa what faith is. He explains that he cannot exactly define the word for her, but that faith is what she exhibits when she sits down in a chair and expects it to hold her up, rather than collapsing and pitching her ass over elbows. That's as good a definition as any, because it uses a real world example to demonstrate what faith is.

Each one of us has a core set of beliefs that we've gathered over the years. These beliefs can be religious in nature (belief in God, Jesus, or Allah), they can be about people (people are generally good / people are generally bad), and they can even be about intangible things (like my belief that diets don't work). Faith is a set of beliefs.

Beliefs are not the same things as truths; make no mistake about that. A belief is not necessarily true; it is merely something we hold to be true, usually based on experience. As with thoughts and words, our beliefs help to mold and determine not only our actions, but also our results. Think about this for a second. If your beliefs affect your actions and your results, can you not change your actions and results by merely changing a particular limiting belief?

Don't tell me it's impossible, because I'm walking and talking proof. I spent 33 years of my life telling myself I was addicted to sugar and eating loads of it daily, until I simply changed my belief with the help of that rotting foot and decided to believe that sugar is poison instead. As a result, I haven't touched sugar in over 10 weeks now, excepting one spoonful of strawberry jam, and I haven't craved it at all. You can change your beliefs instantly, if you simply decide to.

Even Jesus knew the power of belief. He talked about it at great length, as most of history's enlightened teachers have. Remember this one? "With faith (your beliefs) all things are possible." Which things? *All* things. How about "If you had the faith of a mustard seed you could cause a mountain to throw itself into the sea?" Are you starting to see how powerful your beliefs can be?

Let's focus it now on what I'm doing and some of the things I believe and don't believe. I think my actions and results have been fairly outstanding, and I think they are in great part due to my beliefs (or lack of beliefs, in some cases).

- I believe that it's possible to shed weight without being on a "diet."
- I don't believe what I'm doing is "hard," or a "battle," or a "struggle."
- I believe that shedding 183 pounds is easy to do.
- I believe I am 100% healthy, with no signs of diabetes.
- I believe my blood sugar is perfectly normal.
- I don't believe in trying. I believe in doing.
- I don't believe I *can* do this. I believe I *will*.

What do you believe?

August 9

Our thoughts, words, and beliefs can have a tremendous impact on the actions we take to achieve a specific set of results. Most people don't know what results they want when they start out in life. I sure didn't, and I ended up with a 371-pound result that was getting bigger by the day.

Then, in an instant in May, my thoughts transformed from "Little Debbie. Eat. Good," to "Oh my God, I'm going to *die* if I don't do something right now." I made a decision at that point to become fit and healthy. I began to talk like a fit man and believe in my head that I already was fit because I knew that this would immediately start me towards the results I wanted.

As a result of changing my innermost thoughts and beliefs, and modifying my language to remove words like "try," "lose," and "diet," I was able to take massive actions to get to my results. These actions included a complete cessation of sugary food intake; I began to exercise every single day; I started to choose foods that were healthy instead of unhealthy; and I began some serious goal-setting. These actions were and are very powerful for getting me the results I want, and I believe that they're so strong and working so well because of the initial changes I made with the other pieces of the results cycle.

To get the results you want requires a change in the way you do things. The absolute first step is to make a decision to do whatever it takes to get your results. Talk and live as though you're getting your results already. Believe they're attainable and that you have the ability to get them. Follow up with actions, and you're guaranteed success.

August 10

Most people, when you ask them, only have a vague idea of what they want.

"I want to lose weight."

"I need to lose a few pounds."

Stop me. I don't know if I can bear the excitement!

These are the results I'm aiming for: *I will drop 183 pounds over the course of 14 months because I want to live to see my daughter have grandkids of her own. I'll weigh 190 pounds when I finish, I won't have diabetes or any of its symptoms any more, and I'll be medicine free. I'll be able to run miles at a time, and play sports any time I choose without worrying about having a heart attack. I certainly won't be ashamed to go to the beach any more, and I'll fit on all those amusement park rides I've longed to ride.*

And that's just the beginning! I could list pages and pages of results I want, but the ones above sum it up pretty well. Why do I have so many, and why are they so detailed? Because it gets me excited, that's why! Am I more likely to start the results cycle with a vivid and lively set of results or with a single boring one like "I need to lose weight?"

Would you start building a house without a picture of what the final result was going to be? I cannot presume to speak for you, but I want a well-designed house, so I'm going to start with my outcomes clearly labeled and defined.

August 12

Suppose there are three owners of a company, and it comes to their attention that an employee was putting down 8 hours on his timesheet, but wasn't in the office for 8 hours most days. Generally this employee would come in at 8, have an hour for lunch, and leave at 4, giving him a seven-hour day.

Let's listen in on a possible meeting of these owners:

"I think he's made a mistake and believes he gets paid for his lunch time," says Owner 1.

"He knows it's wrong," says Owner 2.

Owner 3 proclaims, "He's lying and he's trying to screw us over."

We have one situation, but three opinions. See how they vary in emotional intensity? While no one response is "right," I do believe if we watch the things we say we can keep in check a lot of the emotions we normally allow to run rampant. I'm not advocating bottling up one's feelings, but I want to show that your words can have a definite effect on your emotional state. To bring it home to the whole weight situation, which phrase below carries the most emotional intensity?

I'm a little hungry.

I'm starving!

If I don't get something to eat soon, I'll die!

What do you think? Is it entirely possible that we can talk ourselves into overeating just by what we tell ourselves about hunger? What about exercise?

It made me a little sore, but it felt good.

I hurt like hell!

I thought I'd never walk again!

While humans aren't quite like Pavlov's dogs, we can condition ourselves by practicing a few different things. One of these is controlling our tongues. The more emotional intensity you have in your words, the more likely you are to link that emotion with whatever action or situation you're talking about.

August 13

In physics, the formula for power is

$$P = \frac{W}{T}$$

where P is power, W is work, and T is time. In words: "Power is work over time." Think about that for a while.

August 14

In every man's life, there comes a time when the proverbial rubber must meet the road. For me, this time came yesterday morning during breakfast. I realized that my posturing and pontificating in this journal was all for naught if I weren't simply willing to put my money where my mouth is and prove once and for all that what I've done in my head has really happened in my body. After all, what good is my newfound faith in myself if I'm not willing to test it, to really stretch my new wings and soar like a dove?

Yesterday I made the decision to stop taking medication for diabetes, against my doctor's wishes. No matter what she says or what the insurance company says, I refuse to believe that I am a diabetic. My blood sugar has been under 100 for the last two months or so, I feel better than I can remember, and I'm tired of popping two pills a day. There's absolutely no chance I'll slip back into my old ways because that man is dead and there's a new one in his place.

Pregnant women who become diabetic during their pregnancy aren't considered life-long diabetics after they give birth. Why then must I have this label attached to me like an albatross around my neck wherever I go? Sure I'm still fat, but I've delivered an unhealthy 64-pound offspring (so far!), and it took the diabetes with it. I am not a diabetic, and I refuse to act like one. You cannot make me, no matter how much you want to.

Take a step back, and watch me fly.

August 15

I made an appointment to have blood work done tomorrow because I want to get my cholesterol and triglycerides checked along with the usual blood sugar counts. If I see my doctor, I'm planning to tell her about my decision to go against her wishes and prove once and for all that I don't have diabetes.

I hope she takes it well.

When I was first diagnosed with Type II diabetes in May of 1997, I pretty much freaked out. My blood sugar at the time was a whopping 403 (for reference, 500 is the low end of diabetic coma levels). My doctor told me of the dangers of this disease, and warned me of a particularly miserable life ahead if I did not mend my wicked ways. The one ray of light she offered was telling me that if I shed my excess weight, I wouldn't be a diabetic any more. She did not say, "It will be controlled." She said, "It will be cured."

Cured. Isn't that a beautiful word? I had within me the whole time the ability to cure myself, only I lacked the faith to let go and just *do* it. On May 28th of this year, I got an abundance of faith, in the form of a diabetic man on television who had to have one leg reduced to a stump because he didn't do the right thing with regards to his health. And people say reality television has no merit.

As some proof in the pudding, for the month or so after my doctor made my diagnosis, I was on a swimming kick, going to a friend's house every afternoon for an hour or so then stopping at Dairy Queen for a blizzard (I told myself I'd *earned* it) on the way home. In June of that same year, when I went back in to have my blood sugar tested it was seventy-four.

Did that wake me up? No. Sometimes I'm a deep sleeper.

By August of that year, I'd stopped swimming and was on Glucophage. We worked with that drug for about 1.5 years, trying all the way up to three pills a day, with no real effect on my blood sugar. Then she switched me to Avandia, first one pill a day, then two. Nothing. Nada. Zilch. The best we ever saw my blood sugar get was in the 130s, but it was usually in the 160s or 170s.

Before my transformation on May 28th, the most previous blood sugar count on her records was from March. It was 199. Fast forward to my test in June, where my blood sugar was 107. Fast forward again, this time to July, where it was 89 – less than two hours after a meal!

Work with me here. Lazy, stuffing my face with sugar, eating wickedly unhealthy food, and taking pills: blood sugar of 199. Changing my beliefs about food, exercising daily, dropping over 60 pounds, not eating sugar, consuming almost exclusively healthy foods, still taking pills: blood sugar of 89.

Forgive me if I don't share the sentiment of my doctor that the pills are what did it.

I checked my blood sugar last night before bed. Once again, it was 89. I'm still planning to check it weekly for the next few months; I'm really not stupid. If I'm wrong, I'll eat crow. I've had it before, and I can stomach the taste.

But I'm not wrong.

August 16

There's a somewhat obscure passage from the book of Proverbs in the Bible. In essence, the quote says, "Without a vision, people perish."

Most people adopt a seat of the pants method when they make the decision to lose weight. I know I sure did for the first several days, when I was riding high on the sight of that rotting foot. It took a little while, but I determined the ultimate outcome I wanted, and designed a simple plan to get that outcome.

Without a vision, people perish.

The biggest reason people fail when they're trying to change is because they don't have a vision. More often, they've decided to lose 10 pounds for a wedding or some event, and the only real plan they make is to follow the fad-diet-of-the-week until they're where they want to be. Sure, it works for the occasional person, but not for very many. It takes a specific vision to make a dream come true.

As I've written so often before, whenever I look in the mirror, I don't see a 309-pound fat man. I see my vision. There's a fit man in there, looking back at me. He's not only fit – he's the very epitome of vibrant health. Physically, he's an Adonis. He's not a diabetic, and there's an almost palpable aura of health around him.

He looks at the world with a sense of wonder, because there are many things he can now do. He can fit on any amusement park ride. He's able to climb flight after flight of stairs without gasping for air or sweating. He can cut his yard in the hottest part of the summer without a problem. He shops for his clothes anywhere he wants, save one store – the Big and Tall shop. He's not embarrassed to go out in public because he no longer feels stared at.

For him, sex has become more fun than ever before, because he doesn't have to stop from tiredness and rest in the middle. Naps are a thing of the past, because he's a bundle of pure energy. As a matter of fact, he cannot even *imagine* taking a nap, because it would take away time from all the fun things he does now. I see him there, gestating now, aching to be born. He waits, patiently, for me to form him and nurture him. He knows that he will be the best thing that ever happened to me, and that I'll love him forever and ever. He's everything I never was.

How can I possibly stop him?

August 17

Having a vision gives you something specific to shoot for, rather than some nebulous, "I need to lose 10 pounds." A vision keeps your dream at the forefront of your thoughts, and makes it difficult, if not even impossible, to fail. If you have a vision, weight reduction is no longer a trial, or a battle, a war, or even particularly difficult. It's just another step in your growth as a person.

Without a vision, you're almost guaranteed to crash and burn.

How then, does one find their vision? All you have to do is look. Think about it. Imagine all the possibilities you have: sickness or health, energy and vitality, the way you want to look and feel, and perhaps the strength you want to have. This is a very personal process, because it's different for each person. Just take the time to think it through, and imagine the impact on every aspect of your life that a new you would have.

- Would you be a better lover?
- Would people look at you when you walk into a room, not because you're so fat, but because you're physically appealing?
- Would you look forward to getting out of bed in the morning?
- Would you be able to shop in a whole new set of stores for clothes?
- What would it be like to only have one chin?
- Would you have any health problems disappear?

Find the vision of the new you, and for goodness' sake, write it down! Most people get a tenuous grasp on a vision for a while, but they don't write it down. Instead, they try to hold it in their head, and invariably forget it, then wonder why the scale's moving the opposite of the way they want it to go.

Put your written vision somewhere where you'll see it daily. Personally, I recommend the bathroom mirror, because we all have to look there pretty much every day. Read it daily, and watch yourself transform.

Who do you want to be today?

August 18

Yesterday I wore a pair of the new 48-inch-waist pants I bought last week, the first time I'd done that this week. Around 9 am, I realized they were dropping down on my butt whenever I stood up. Not that I'm complaining. Turns out I needed to move in another hole on the belt. The 52-inch pants I still wear were just bunching up so I didn't notice the need to tighten it up.

But that's not the best part, not at all.

When I got home from work, I strutted around like a peacock, showing my wife how my belt needed to really be on the next hole. When I went upstairs to change clothes so I could go clean the pool, I took off my belt and headed for the closet for something more casual.

And my new 48-inch-waist pants fell off.

Suppose there's a person you know. This person, whom we'll arbitrarily make male, sees something in life that he wants more than anything. He thinks it through, and makes a decision to get what he wants. He creates a vision of his dream, and writes it down to study regularly. He sets a specific goal, along with a goal date, of when he wants to have his dream.

His reasons are compelling, and he has them all written down so he can review them consistently. He's set milestones along the way to achieving this dream, and he checks them off as he passes them. There may be some trials along the way, but his eye is on the future, and he sees nothing other than what he has chosen to obtain. He is fully dedicated to making this dream come true, and will let nothing stand in his way.

He's relentless in his pursuit of this dream, and never once questions whether or not he will achieve it. Others have tried before him and failed. Their remains litter his path, and they serve as a reminder to him what can happen if he ever loses his focus. It takes time to make the dream come true, but he understands that as long as he stands strong, and lets nothing cloud his vision, nothing can stop the dream.

Achieving the dream has been likened to a long journey. Many view the journey to be too difficult, and give up along the way. Worse yet, some give up without even trying. This man is different, because his plan is different, and for him the journey is not difficult. The journey, for this man, is just a means for making his dream come true. He cannot waver, because he sees only his dream.

Finally, the man reaches the end of his journey, and holds the thing he once only dreamed about. Success is his, and he can stand tall, and remember the things he went through to get this dream. His life is overflowing with abundance, because his dream has come true through his determination, effort, and patience.

Why, then, do we call this man "lucky?"

August 19

Today, after running errands, I went by a local fitness equipment store and picked out a big home gym so I can start weight training, because I intend on not merely being fit, but being buff.

Now I just need to convince my wife to let me buy it.

August 20

In ophthalmology, retinal or optical nerve damage or degeneration can cause a condition known as a *scotoma*. Specifically, this is an area of decreased vision that can make it difficult to do things like read or watch TV, because you cannot clearly see the things directly in front of the area. More commonly, a scotoma is called a "blind spot."

It's entirely possible to create your own scotoma. Have you ever been looking in the refrigerator, and been asked to get something out, perhaps the Tabasco sauce, while you're there? You mumble to yourself, "I don't know where the dang Tabasco sauce is," and skim the contents of the refrigerator.

"It's not here!" you proclaim, then watch as your friend or spouse comes over and takes it right out from under your nose, giving you a dirty look.

Was the Tabasco there? Yes. Did your eyes see it? Yes. What happened? You created a scotoma by initially telling yourself you couldn't see the Tabasco sauce. Your brain was merely obliging you.

For the first 33 years of my life, almost to the day, I had a huge scotoma that kept me from clearly seeing what I was doing to myself. The worst part about this scotoma is that I caused it, because I constantly told myself things like, "I'm fat, but I'm not *real* fat," and "Diabetes won't hurt me while I'm young, I can just straighten out my eating later."

Sure enough, when I'd look at myself in the mirror, I was pretty happy. I knew that I was a big guy, and I felt uncomfortable around people because I thought they stared at me, but I thought everything was okay, because that's what I told myself. Having a blood sugar level 60 points above the high end of normal was okay, because heck, it's still less than 200, right?

Thanks to an enlightening vacation followed by a television show, my scotoma disappeared, and for the first time in my life I saw myself with absolute clarity. I saw a man who was pushing 400 pounds and was a heart attack in waiting. His face wasn't recognizable because it was stretched so far out of proportion. He had fat packed all over him, and he was trying to pack even more on. His stomach sagged several inches, and he had breasts bigger than most women.

Clear vision can help you work miracles on yourself. As I write this, my stomach only sags about an inch now, and I assume when the sag goes it'll start flattening out. When I stand and move either my arms or legs, I can see muscles underneath sliding and rippling. My calves are actually cut, and have some nice definition. My boobs are still big, but now they're perky.

August 21

I took my daughter bowling yesterday. The good news is that my arm feels great today. The bad news is that I apparently pulled my left butt cheek. I wasn't aware that was possible. Luckily, it didn't prevent me from riding the stationary bike this morning. I'm thinking of setting a mini-goal to have at least one day where no part of me is hurting.

❧

The only way to make any sort of significant change in your life is to raise your standards. When it comes to our health, why do we accept anything but the very best? We keep low standards for our bodies, then we wonder how we end up (in my case) weighing almost 400 pounds, with diabetes.

Think about it for a second – how long did you spend planning your last vacation? How many hours deciding where to go, where to stay, whether to drive or fly, and what you wanted to do while there? I cannot speak for anyone but myself here – I spent at least 5 hours just trying to find a place to stay back when we visited Gatlinburg in May.

How much time do you spend planning for your health? Often, we go through life as though we're just along for the ride, rather than working on a design for our bodies and our health. The standards we have for our health are abysmally low, or nonexistent. Why do we do so much less than we're capable of? Worse yet, we make up excuses that invariably blame external sources for our lack of high standards.

Consider a typical health-related question: *Why don't you exercise regularly?*

"It makes me too tired."

"I don't have time because I work, and go to school."

"I don't have the energy because I'm (insert malady here)."

If you want to merely get by in life, these are all fine reasons for not exercising. However, if you want to design a life full of energy and vitality, you have to raise your standards, and decide that you will exercise, whatever it takes. For me, taking a shower every morning is not an option; it's just something I do. Exercise is the exact same. There's no "if" about exercising for me.

The same thing goes for eating. Before May of this year, I didn't really care what I ate or how much. Since then, I've raised my standards and no longer eat many of the foods I once considered staples. Chief among these is sugary stuff. Additionally, I don't eat much fried food or as much red meat, and I've cut white flour almost completely. Instead, I choose more chicken, fish, and vegetables. Ninety percent or more of the grains I eat are whole, and not processed. In short, I've changed these things because I have a new set of standards, and they're reshaping my life.

What are your standards?

August 22

I ordered a home gym today so I can start lifting weights.

Most attempts to shed weight or become healthy through sheer willpower are doomed to fail. I realize that statement puts a lot of people on the defensive because most people have very deeply held beliefs about willpower. Regardless, this is one of the main reasons that long term dieting is almost guaranteed to not be successful. Most likely you grew up with beliefs about the strength of willpower, programmed with phrases like "fake it till you make it," and these ideas set a vicious trap.

In most instances of willpower, one desire you have is directly opposed to another. For example, it might be something like the desire to be thin versus the desire to eat a bag of cookies. By using willpower to deny the cookie desire, you suppress that desire with the stronger one.

This works for a while, then guess what happens? You suppress and suppress and suppress the call of the Oreos until a day comes when the desire for the Oreos overcomes the desire to be thin. And then you binge and eat a whole bag in one sitting, rather than the two or three you would've normally eaten. You beat yourself to death with guilt and proclaim to people around you that you "have no willpower."

What generally happens here is one of two things. Either you give up, or you try again only to have the same results. Neither path leads to success. It teaches you that you cannot win; that you're a failure. It shows everyone around you that you're inconsistent, and eventually reduces you to a point of burnout where you don't even want to try.

I've found out a great secret. The trick is to find a way to completely remove the desire for the Oreos, so you don't have to worry about will power.

August 23

This morning I weighed, for the first time since 1992 – not counting the brief instance in 1995 – less than 300 pounds. I was so happy I thought I was going to cry. I even weighed myself three times to make sure it wasn't a fluke, and at no time did the scales ever cross the 300 mark.

I didn't really want to write about this, because my weight fluctuates quite a bit during the week, and I'm not positive it will stay below 300 over the next few days. It's a little funny, because for the last three months I've considered myself a fairly motivated person with regards to getting the fat gone and being a healthy man. I was wrong. My motivation before was a mere shadow to what I have now.

Two things motivate every human – regardless of age, sex, weight, race, or religion. You can call them pain and pleasure, comfort and discomfort, joy and sorrow, agony and ecstasy, or love and hate. My personal preference is call them pain and pleasure.

Specifically, we're motivated to move away from anything that brings us what we perceive as pain, and toward anything that brings us what we perceive as pleasure. This pain or pleasure can be mental, emotional, spiritual, physical, or any combination of these.

I call the technique for eliminating desires "finding your pain." When you find it, you know it, because the desire for something not only just goes away, that very thing becomes repugnant. It's not a magic trick, and it's not willpower. It changes you at your most basic level.

Finding your pain means to find just one thing, no matter how big or small, that makes life as you know it so painful, so unbearable, that it becomes impossible to keep doing things the way you're doing them now. I wish I could offer a panacea that worked for everyone, but finding your pain is a very personal thing.

My pain, as you already know, was coming to the realization that unless I took immediate action, I was destined to spend my life in an ever-declining state of health that included kidney failure, amputations, blindness, and ultimately death at a young age. Mine was a pretty major pain, to say the least. Yours may be different, but until you find a way to make the pain massive, you're not going to be able to make a real change in your life.

Once you've found your pain, you begin to realize you're looking at the world through a new set of eyes – the eyes of a changed person. The names Ben and Jerry suddenly mean nothing. Oreos are just artery-clogging poison, and Little Debbie is just some tramp displaying her goodies everywhere. You don't have to quash a desire, because the desire is gone.

My wife, Robyn, found her pain a couple of months ago, when she was parking at the grocery store. Just as she was about to get out of her car, she saw a very large older woman walking up to the store to buy more food. The woman could barely walk and was wincing with every step she took. Robyn's pain was coming to the understanding that her future was going to be like that, full of aches and pains that she could prevent if only she wanted to. I'm pleased to say that as of today, Robyn has dropped over 30 pounds.

Think about your life. Find your pain.

August 24

Last night, after I'd written about how happy I was to weigh less than 300 pounds, Robyn told me she'd found a bottle cap under the scales, throwing off the reading by two pounds. Damn. If nothing else, it was fun while it lasted. I guess it was a bit of a pipe dream to think I'd dropped a couple of pounds overnight, huh?

I'll just cross 300 again next week, for real.

August 25

My gym machine was delivered today, and I'm a little torn as to whether to start using it yet or to wait another 50-60 pounds as originally planned.

I'm concerned that if I start lifting weights now, and cut my aerobic stuff back to 3 or 4 times a week, I'll sabotage the speed at which I'm throwing weight off. According to one of my friends, and the guy who set this machine up (he was once a personal trainer), I can use this machine aerobically by using low weights and lifting them quickly. I don't know; I need to think about it a bit.

This leads to my thoughts for tonight. My concern over slowing the weight shedding concerns me. When I started out to get my life into shape, fat liberation was a side effect of becoming healthy. Over the last month or so, however, my focus has moved more to getting the weight down, with the health thing becoming more of a side effect. I believe this is merely because the weight shedding is the most visible aspect of becoming healthy, but I'm not completely sure. If my focus were still truly on becoming healthy, I wouldn't be so concerned about the weight issue.

It took my wife to point this out to me, and for her perspective I am eternally grateful. I won't lie, I am very interested in getting the weight down, and I may leave that as my focus, because getting the weight down cannot help but make me healthier. Does that make sense?

The main reason I'm a bit concerned about the weight shedding slowing down is this: at my current weight I can burn some hellacious calories when I do my aerobic workout. I think it's in my best interest to take advantage of that.

August 27

According to an article I just read, every additional pound of muscle mass you have can increase your metabolism by as much as 50 calories per day.

Therefore, after much deliberation, talking to the wife, two personal trainers, and soliciting the opinions of people around the world via email, I have decided to begin weight training tomorrow. I'll be training with weights on Monday, Wednesday, and Friday, and some form of cardio work on the other days of the week.

I anticipate serious pain for the next few weeks.

August 29

I was sore today, but not terribly so. It didn't take anything but a little stretching to get me ready for 20 minutes on the stationary bike. I think

I reached a new high intensity there, because I burned almost as many calories in 20 minutes as I normally do in 30.

I was pretty tired most of the day. I think the combination of a higher intensity workout and the amount of work I now put my muscles through may call for an earlier bedtime. I'll try tonight and see what happens. Tomorrow morning is weights again, only this time I'm working on my lower body. My intentions are to work pretty hard on my abs, but I haven't decided on my legs because after all, these legs have already been carrying around almost 400 pounds for the last several years.

August 31

Over the last couple of days, I've been giving my weight training some thought, and I've reached a conclusion: I am going to stop weight training until I reach a considerably lower weight, like 220 or 230 pounds.

Call me vain, call me unfocused, or call me a wimp. I set a goal for myself that I gave myself till next July to reach. I take my goals very seriously, and while I now believe 190 pounds is going to be a bit light for the amount of muscle bulk I want to have (I'm thinking more like 200). I will make the date. Of that I am certain.

And herein lies the rub. While weight training this week, between Monday and today, my weight dropped exactly 1/2 pound. Yes, I'm aware that any move in the positive is welcome, but I normally have dropped two or three pounds by this time in the week. It would appear that my concerns of last week might be valid: the weight training is not aerobic, and neither is the intense stationary bike riding, so I'm burning up glycogen rather than fat.

I'm sure my liver loves me for it.

Perhaps I am obsessed too much by the weight, but like I said before, meeting a goal is very important to me. Weight training is not a matter of if, just a matter of when, and when is going to be in another 70 or 80 pounds.

As things stand, I shall return to my daily aerobic routine starting tomorrow. Only now I guess I can stare longingly at my home gym while I do it.

September 2000

300 – 288 *pounds*

September 3

I learned a great truth this morning when I got out of bed. I realized that walking for real and walking with videotapes are far from being the same. Yesterday, I decided to walk outside for the first time since I started exercising, and I walked for an hour. I went 3.3 miles.

It wouldn't be so bad if the pain confined itself to my legs, but my back hurts too, all the way up to my shoulder blades. My lower back hurts the most; it actually aches even when I'm not doing anything, but really flares up when I get up and walk around. Perhaps I was a little too active yesterday.

In addition to the 3.3 miles of actual real-world walking, I went up to Tennessee and traipsed around Mennonite country, I went swimming last night, and I performed sexual gymnastics on three separate occasions with my wife yesterday.

No wonder I hurt today.

When I was super-fat, as opposed to the really-fat that I am now, I had to take an acid-blocker every night before bed to keep me from waking up with bad heartburn in the middle of the night. It was so bad some nights that I'd wake up unable to breathe because I'd started to vomit up acid in my sleep. Nothing's quite as frightening as popping out of a dead sleep and not being able to breathe. When I stopped taking my diabetes medicine a few weeks ago, I also stopped taking my nightly acid-blocker pill, and I'm pleased to tell you that I've not had heartburn once.

This fat liberation thing just keeps getting better and better.

September 5

I weigh less than 300 pounds now. Officially.

For the last month or so, I've been a little troubled. Have you ever wondered if you'll miss the fat version of you when you're thin? When I use the word "miss," I don't mean it in the sense of having a desire to be back there, but more like a wistful fondness. Sort of a nostalgic feeling towards the way things once were. After dropping this 74 pounds, I already feel like a different person. I look considerably different today than I did just a few short months ago, and I'll continue to change physically over the next several months. Seeing this new Fred in the mirror is a little like looking at a stranger sometimes.

Don't get me wrong. I like the new Fred, like him a lot, but the physical changes I've wrought in myself have taken me way out of what was once my comfort zone. It's a little intimidating at times. He doesn't scare me; he just keeps me on my toes and makes me think fondly of the days when I was fat and happy.

When I look at this new man in the mirror I not only see a face with an actual shape, I even see a neck. This new man has large man-boobs, only his are nice and perky instead of sagging practically to his belly button. His gut is large, but like the man-boobs, it merely pokes out, no longer drooping over his genitals. The man I see when I look in the mirror has some cut to his legs, and he can feel his ribs when he lies in the bed at night with his wife.

I like to look at this man in the mirror. Like it a lot, I do, even to the point of being chastised for narcissism by my wife. She's beginning to understand a bit, I think, because she's noticing a new Robyn these days. Now she understands my obsession with this man, at least a little. He interests me to no end because of all the things about him (in a physical sense) I can now see that I'd forgotten.

Know what the best part is about seeing this new man? I haven't seen *anything* yet.

September 7

We live in an ever-increasingly busy society, and it seems like everyone wants a piece of our time. Have you noticed this? We get so busy doing things for everyone else that we forget to take time for the most important person in our lives – ourselves. We please others and stress ourselves out.

Stop and take time for yourself each day. The world won't stop spinning. Get away from the needs and wants of everyone around you and have some quiet time just for yourself. Some people might tell you you're selfish, but that's okay. If you want a happy and successful life, you have to take time for yourself. One thing I've found is that my morning exercise time gives me ample opportunities to disengage my brain from what I'm doing, and just reflect on life. Four-thirty in the morning is a pretty quiet time, which is perfect for introspection.

I think about all sorts of things then – things I'm grateful for, how I'm changing my body for the better, my mood, and my overall happiness. Taking this time each morning really sets the speed for the whole day, and fills me with almost boundless joy and energy. Take care of yourself first, and you can better serve those around you.

September 10

I was reminded yesterday of the frailty of human life, while I sat in the funeral home with my extended family. My second cousin Jeffrey died on Wednesday afternoon, and we were gathered together to bury him. Jeffrey was twelve years old.

Nothing brings home how precious life is like the death of a child, and it raised in me some very serious questions. Why do we spend so much time being unhappy when our lives can end in a split second? Why do we focus so much on doing things we don't want to do when we know beyond the shadow of a doubt that we're going to die? Why don't we enjoy life more?

We waste our lives, and make the most special gift in the world into a mockery. God knows I did my share. I spent the last several years wasting the life that had been given to me. I'd become a prisoner, ashamed to go out in public because I weighed nearly 400 pounds. My wife and I never did much together outside the house because I was so fat that people stared at us. I deprived myself of having fun for eight years, and deprived my wife and child for almost four.

No more.

Even if I did manage to get out, like our trip to Gatlinburg in May, I was limited in what I could do because of my size. Do you know what it's like to have to tell your child you cannot go on the "Earthquake" ride because the seatbelt won't go around you? How about not being able to go on the virtual roller coaster ride because it has a 480-pound weight limit, and after subtracting your weight there's only about 100 pounds left over? What about wanting to hike that nature trail in the Smoky Mountains but not doing it because you were afraid you'd get out in the woods and not be able to walk the whole trail?

No more.

If this life is worth having, then by God it's worth living to its absolute fullest.

September 12

When you rationalize, you're attributing your actions to creditable motives without really giving any thought to what the unconscious motives are. I used to spend a lot of time rationalizing being so fat to myself.

I'm not really that big. After all, the pants in the fat man's store went up to sixty inches, and I was in a comfortable 54. Hell, I had a couple more sizes to work through before I really needed to worry.

You're not really a diabetic unless your fasting blood sugar is over 200, I told myself, reading the measurement in the 180s off my Glucometer.

That Earthquake ride in Gatlinburg? It probably sucked anyway. It didn't matter that the seatbelt wouldn't go around me.

I love flying first class. Being embarrassed at the thought of drooping over into the next seat next or having to ask the attendant for a seatbelt extender had nothing to do with it.

I was lying my way to an early grave. Fortunately, I found a little truth serum a few months back, and the lies are gone now. Have you been lying to yourself?

September 16

Recently, I was asked why I set such a monumental goal for shedding weight, rather than setting smaller, possibly more manageable goals. I'd like to share my thoughts on this.

For me, a goal is a destination, a final ending place. If I set a goal to drop 20 pounds, where's the incentive to drop 20 more? I've reached my goal, and now I have to set a new one. Personally, I'd rather achieve the goal I want, and move on to something else. If I sit around telling myself (assuming a 20-pound goal) "all I have to drop is 10 more pounds," then I'm not only trying to fool myself, I'm making it easier to fail, because I don't need to drop 20 pounds, I need to drop almost 200. When I reach that 20-pound goal, I feel like I can quit.

I'm no quitter.

Instead of setting small goals, I imagine my weight marked off on a line, from 373 to 190 counting downwards from left to right. On this line, I see specific weights, which I consider milestones to be passed, not goals to be reached. Let me share some of my markers:

The first marker on my weight line was 350 pounds, because that meant I could once again be weighed on normal doctor's scales. Next was 329, because that's one pound less than the weight I held for several years in the mid-90s. 300 was marked, because it was a magical round number, of course.

The next one I'm looking forward to hitting is 288, because it's one pound less than the weight I reached when I dropped 50 pounds back in 1995 and it's right around the corner. After that, 271 marks the 100-pound mark. 258 puts me one pound under where I was when I graduated from college in 1990. The round numbers 250, 225, and 200 are marked, too.

Finally, my last marker is 196, because that's what I weighed when I graduated from high school in 1985. I'm really hoping to hit this, but to be completely honest, I'm not sure if I will because of the weight training I'm planning in 40 or 50 more pounds.

But really, which is more important: the final number on a scale or my health?

September 22

In a recent email, someone told me my weight results (84 pounds in 116 days and counting) were not typical, which makes me think of a diet commercial. In my response, I commented that my results were typical, but my approach to shedding the weight wasn't. This is something I believe with all my heart.

I regularly read people's diet journals on the web, and check out message boards online almost daily. Things I seem to see a lot are emotional eating, bingeing, and progress reports that would look like a cross-section of the ocean if graphed, waves and all. When I read more closely, I find that most of the unsuccessful people are looking at this whole process of becoming fit/healthy in a decidedly unhealthy light.

There are a couple of adages that are very important to having a total transformation from chunk to hunk. Specifically, they're "attitude is everything" and "your attitude determines your altitude." As a matter of fact, not only do I think they're merely important, I think they are of paramount importance, because with the wrong attitude, you're doomed either to fail outright, or to wade in a cyclic 5-pound limbo virtually forever.

I have nothing to hide in dropping 84 pounds so fast. I'm doing, in a physical sense, what a lot of people before me have done. I'm eating less than I used to and I'm moving a whole lot more. I'm not starving by any stretch of the imagination, and I'm not exercising myself into the ground. Exercise and diet are important, sure, because you cannot simply think yourself thin, as much as we might want to. It takes a little bit of action.

September 23

As I said yesterday, I believe attitude is the most important piece in the weight-loss puzzle, because I believe that the human brain can do most anything it wants. If it wants a 98-pound mother to lift a car off her trapped child, it will make it happen. If it wants a 371-pound man to drop nearly 200 pounds in 14 months, it will make it happen. And if your brain gets a notion for you to drop the weight you want gone in a certain time frame, it can make that happen, too.

The fourth definition of the word "attitude," according to the dictionary, is "a mental position with regard to fact or state." Notice that attitude deals with both facts (truths) and states (an emotional atmosphere). Your attitude is simply your outlook towards these. Suppose the following statements sum up a person's attitude about shedding weight:

"It's so hard for me to lose weight."

"When I try to lose weight, I starve all the time."

"I can't lose weight, because I have no self-control."

The list goes on and on. Would you say these statements display a good attitude or a bad attitude? I contend they show a negative attitude, what I call the "I can't" attitude. You set yourself up for failure talking like this, because you program yourself to do so.

If you believe something, then for you that thing will become true.

How about these:

"I'm trying to lose weight."

"I think I can do it."

You already know what I think about the words "try" and "can." They're products of the wrong kind of attitude for success. Perhaps I sound a bit arrogant, and perhaps I *am* a bit arrogant, but I don't believe in merely trying to do something. Either do it, or don't do it. Don't try. If you don't get the results you want, change your approach and do it again.

And don't say you think you can do something. Of course you can, because you have the ability to do anything you set your mind to doing. "Can" is another reason to fail.

People regularly tell me how surprised they are that I'm dropping weight so fast. Why? I said I was going to, and I focused completely on doing it. I explain everything I do – my eating, my exercise, and my thought processes – and still people are surprised. When I went off my diabetes medicine, the naysayers came out and told me how wrong I was, because they apparently know more about my body than I do. I've been off the medicine now for 5 weeks with no problems, and continue to have normal blood-sugar levels.

It may sound arrogant, but my point is simply this: believe totally in yourself, and don't let anyone drag you down with his or her beliefs. Focus completely and positively on where you want to be, and don't waver. If you believe whole-heartedly that you will do something and take the actions necessary to do it, then you'll do it. Don't give your brain the option of failing, and you'll not fail. Even if you miss your goal slightly, you're guaranteed to get considerably further with the right attitude than with the wrong one.

September 25

I must admit it. I'm stumped. Confused, perplexed, and astounded. Something I never expected would happen has happened, several times now, and I'm still trying to figure out how and why.

The first time it happened, I thought it was an anomaly. The second time, I wrote it off as stress. The third time, I became curious. And when it happened the fourth time, just today, I felt the first pangs of concern. Not major pangs, but some definite minor ones. Twinges, really, but twinges nonetheless.

I'm talking about the most surprising thing that's happened to me in the last four months – something I've not encountered yet, as I said. I must admit I've even gotten cocky about it, standing proudly on my imagined mountain and smiling gleefully down on all the weak people. Knowing in my heart I'd never have to deal with anything so common, because my way was the best way, and if people would just listen to me, they'd see the light and join me on the mountain.

Apparently I was wrong, because...

I've been having serious cravings over the last several days.

It happened first on Saturday morning, while I was in the grocery store. I was in the store later than normal, around 9:00, and I hadn't had breakfast yet. Rounding the turn into the candy aisle, I was presented with an array of sweets stretching away before me. I had to buy Robyn some Tic-Tacs, which brought me to a stop in front of the candy. Finding them was easy enough, and as I stepped back to my cart, the candy bars – Snickers in particular – caught my eye. It was as though a demon suddenly possessed me, and I found myself lusting over the Snickers bars. I had to face this demon alone, sort of a modern day Van Helsing, if you will.

I found myself strolling the remaining aisles in the store, thinking constantly about buying a single candy bar and eating it in the car alone before I went home. The worst part was that I knew it was pathetic, and I didn't care. That knowledge wasn't going to stop me. Nor would the knowledge that I wasn't starving, that I would be eating a nice healthy breakfast as soon as I got home. You know what the one thing was that kept me from buying the Snickers bar, from crouching in my car like some sort of seedy porn character and eating it furtively, eyes cutting back and forth as though I were breaking a law?

I'd like to say it was something noble, like having a moment of epiphany where I realized that I was more powerful than any simple urge, but I'd be lying if I did. The simple fact of the matter is this: I was afraid my wife would smell the chocolate on my breath and root out my secret. That she'd realize I was no superman at all, but rather a mere mortal who couldn't control himself when dealing with a tiny (albeit unexpected) little urge.

So I left the candy bar on the shelf and went home to my breakfast, a bowl of Total.

Later in that same day, I had my second urge. While not nearly as powerful as the first, this is the one I gave in to. When lunchtime rolled around I found myself in the kitchen looking for something to eat, but not finding anything appealing. What I wanted more than sandwiches was fast food, Taco Bell in particular.

I stalked around the house for a good fifteen minutes, growing more and more agitated at my inability to decide on what to have for lunch. Finally, I said "to hell with it" to myself, and trucked down to the border, where I ordered a formerly normal meal. The upside to this event is that I ended up eating only about half of what I ordered, and threw the rest away because I was so stuffed.

September 27

I had the strong and sudden urge for Snickers candy bars again Sunday, only this time I wanted a whole six-pack instead of a single bar. Fortunately I was unable to convince my wife to pick some up while she was out running errands, and so another craving was stymied.

The last and quite possibly the strongest of the urges hit me Monday afternoon while I was preparing spaghetti for dinner. I was looking in the pantry for the angel hair when a bag of chocolate chips caught my eye. I stared at the bag for some time, debating whether or not to have some. Ultimately, I decided not to have the chocolate chips, and finished cooking dinner.

September 30

After going for almost four months without any real cravings, I must admit I thought I really and truly had that issue licked. I thought I was different, that I'd unlocked a secret that had been lost through the ages. When they showed up last week I was a little confused, to say the least, and somewhat panicked because I figured it would just be a matter of time, given my ideas on willpower and how it doesn't work.

My first thoughts were that the cravings were related, in some way, to the final vestiges of the diabetes medicine working out of my system. In the documentation for that medication it says it takes 8 to 12 weeks to begin working at its fullest potential, so I figured it may very well take that long to work its way completely out.

The second idea I had, which was far and away the most frightening, was that I had lost my pain, my moving force. Remember that lovely gangrenous foot, the result of a life of not caring about diabetes and its side effects that started it all for me? My thoughts went something like this:

What if (all the *really* bad questions start with those two words) *I've gotten content now that I've dropped over 80 pounds? The diabetes is gone, and if I just stay at this weight, I won't have to worry about losing any limbs or dying from diabetes-related complications. What if I've stopped caring at a deep level? Will I have to find some new mental pain to keep me going?*

My third inclination, more likely closer to correct than my first two, is that in every instance of a craving I was also physically hungry. Since sweet foods were one of my biggest downfalls in my old life, a craving for such was inevitable at some point. Old habits die hard.

I'm pretty sure I killed the cravings yesterday. When I walked into work, the first thing I saw was a birthday cake on our conference table, left over from a birthday celebration on Thursday. Ironically, I sat through the whole little party without wanting any cake at all, but when I saw it yesterday, I wanted a piece, and I wanted it bad.

Rather than suppress this craving, I opened the cake box and cut myself a piece. Deprivation, after all, will ultimately lead to failure. I simply decided this time to eat some cake, not go overboard, and enjoy it so I wouldn't feel deprived. I took the first bite of cake, mouth watering and with my eyes closed, and found it awful.

It was cloyingly sweet, and burned my throat almost to the point of making my eyes water. The icing was thick and sludgy, and greased up the inside of my mouth. I imagined it lining my arteries and slowing the flow of blood to a crawl, a thought that sickened me almost as much as the burning sweetness had. I put the fork down, my craving vanquished.

Over the last four months my body has grown accustomed to not only *not* eating sweet foods but also to having almost 100% of what I put into it actually be good for it. As a result, eating the bite of cake was a bit, I suppose, like eating some rat poison, and it disgusted me accordingly. I'm pretty sure that I've seen the last of those sugar cravings for a while now.

October 2000

287 – 281 *pounds*

October 5

I've looked over the family tree, and I don't see any particular branches that droop a little lower than those around them, or that grow leaves a bit slower than the others. Why then do I seem to have such a gift for stupidity? Regularly I amaze myself at the idiotic things I can do, all the while thinking I'm one smart cookie.

For a couple of weeks I've been burning with a strange new desire – a desire that, in retrospect, was stupid to give into. I felt this desire pulling at me most mornings while walking through the neighborhood, listening to an audio book and tromping along fat and happy. Yesterday, I made my big mistake that got me in the jam I'm in right now.

Instead of taking the next audio book CD with me for my walk, I took a CD of upbeat, happy songs, because I thought a little music would make for a welcome change. I was just about to leave the main road I was walking on to go back into the subdivision where I live, when the audio book disc ended. I put in the music CD, pressed the play button, and as I crossed the street, the music began to play. The urge hit as the song began, and it hit hard. Almost against my will I succumbed to it, powerless to resist or fight it in any way.

I started running.

Not power walking, not jogging. Running. Almost a sprint, and I did it for close to a quarter of a mile before the pain in my left foot brought me back to a walk. I can only imagine how I must've looked, bounding down the road like the Michelin Man. I thank God that it was still dark outside, so no one could see me.

The pounding I could feel throughout my body with each step was substantial. From my feet all the way to my head, I could feel it snapping tendons and grinding bones, but I kept going, not quite a runner's "high" but feeling really good. The desire to run had been with me for several days, but I never ran because I knew it would be a real beating on my body.

I received payment in spades this morning for yesterday's debacle. I'm sore up both legs (particularly my left quadriceps) to a degree, and quite sore up my back. Oddly, I never imagined running would make the muscles in my back sore. I can only guess that it's related to the flailing of my arms while I ran. These pains aren't really that bad, and I can get rid of them just by stretching the muscles a little, though they come back after a few moments of inactivity.

The real pain is in my right ankle, which gets worse the more I use it, rather than better. As a result of this pain, I only made it 0.6 miles this morning, before having to turn around and hobble home. That trip, which would normally take me about 20 minutes (round trip, I mean), took about 35 today because I had to walk so slowly. I'm hoping that if I take it easy the rest of today, I'll be able to walk again tomorrow for my normal 2.6 miles (an odd number, I know, but it takes exactly 45 minutes).

October 8

I noticed, yesterday while I was admiring myself shirtless in the mirror, as I so often do, that my gut has tiny wrinkles across it at the bottom. Little ones, and they're there because my skin is now officially too big for my shrinking belly. Imagine a latex helium balloon that you've kept around long enough for it to stop floating and shrink down almost to its uninflated size. Know how the balloon gets all wrinkly because it's gotten too stretched out of shape? That's how my belly is, to a very minor extent.

It would appear that even though the pounds are dropping slowly right now, things are still rearranging themselves in my body. In the last three weeks I've only dropped about 7 pounds, but my 46-inch pants have gone from snug and tight to sliding down my ass while I walk, if I'm not wearing a belt. They won't fall off on their own now, but they're getting close.

I sure can make myself sound sexy.

October 13

I've been reflecting on my new life today, and would like to share. I've exercised for 118 straight days now, something I never imagined doing. I can zip up the stairs now without having any increase at all in my breathing, and there's no longer a pounding of blood in my ears. I've been off diabetes medicine for almost two months, and still have perfectly normal blood sugar. As a result of normal blood sugar, I no longer get large and painful boils all over my body.

I've shed the equivalent of three hundred fifty six sticks of butter, or ten gallons of water, or an 8- or 9-year-old child from my body. I've dropped almost 1/4 of my original total body weight. My waist has shrunk seven inches, and I've dropped two whole X's off my shirt size. I can exercise 45 straight minutes without being sore. I can run again. I've under-grown one belt, and am on the last hole of my newest belt.

I can maintain an erection almost indefinitely now, whereas previously that was just a dream. As long as I'm on that subject, certain parts of my body have gotten larger. Either that or it just looks bigger relative to the rest of me.

I no longer take daily naps, though I snoozed in my big comfy chair today. I sleep the whole night through, most nights. Heartburn is a thing of the past. I no longer have to take a Zantac, Pepcid, or Tagamet before bed. I no longer snore. Goodbye to that sleep apnea, too, while I'm at it. I haven't been sick since I changed my eating habits. Before, I got bronchitis pretty much every three months or less.

I feel about ten years younger these days. I can do pushups again. I can squat. I can get up from the floor without grabbing onto a piece of furniture for help. My belly no longer rubs the steering wheel in my Jeep, and the seatbelt doesn't make me feel uncomfortable any more, because it no longer draws attention to the size of my man-boobs. I don't make the bedroom floor creak nearly as much when I walk across it. My blood pressure is down almost 20 points, both on systolic and diastolic. Seeing the Fred I want to be, when I look in the mirror, gets easier with each passing day, because I'm looking more and more like him. I'm no longer embarrassed to go out in public.

I could go on and on, but I'll stop here. I ended up writing more than I intended, but it's hard to stop once you really open up to the incredible changes that have taken place within you. I can only imagine what I'll be like when I drop the next 89.

If ever you've dreamed of dropping your excess weight, I can think of no better reasons than any of the ones I listed above. If I could share with you for just ten seconds how I feel today compared to how I felt back in May, I would. If I could just give you a taste, no matter how small, of how things are now, I would. You'd never be the same.

October 15

I went to Walmart yesterday and bought a mountain bike. It really is true, by the way. You don't forget how to ride. I rode for seven miles this morning, and loved every minute of it.

Of course, I don't love the achy bruised feeling between my legs at the base of my butt cheeks. That particular pain tends to flare up whenever I sit down. And to be honest, I don't love the muscle ache in my middle back that I'm sure I picked up as part of the overall stabilization process of keeping me balanced for those seven miles.

But all the pain is worth the pleasure of feeling the wind on my face, feeling the muscles in my legs working to zoom me down the road. I wouldn't trade that feeling for anything, especially not for something as trivial as a little ache in my muscles. God knows I've gotten used to that.

I'm not going to stop my jog-walking, not at all, but in deference to my knees and ankles I'm only planning to jog-walk three or four times a week now, and probably cycle the other days, weather permitting. Ironically, one of my friends has been trying to talk me into buying a mountain bike, but I've been mostly against it because I figured it would be hard to keep a close eye on the sidewalk when it's still dark outside. My daughter, however, has decided she wants a new bike for her birthday and that got me to thinking about how much I enjoyed riding in my youth, so

I bought one, too.

❧

Yesterday morning, while I was making breakfast, my daughter came up to me from behind and wrapped her arms around my gut to hug me. That's not unusual at all, but this time something registered in my head as not being quite right. I was measuring oatmeal when she did it, and the wrongness of the hug didn't jibe with me until she was pulling away.

I put down the measuring cup and asked her to come do it again. She did, and I watched down my front as her hands came around me. During the hug she was able to interlock her hands together easily, whereas just a few months ago, her fingertips wouldn't even touch.

Add that one to my list of special things from my last entry.

October 17

When bulls are being trained for bullfighting events in Spain, they are pricked with swords again and again. The bulls are then rated according to their willingness to come back to fight after each wound is inflicted.

If you pick up an axe, and take a swing at a 100-year-old oak tree in the front yard, there will be no real effect on the tree. But, if you do that same thing over and over thousands of times even the biggest tree will eventually fall.

Spawning salmon swim up waterfalls. Surely you've seen the videos on public television or one of the nature channels where bears stand by the stream and catch the fish out of the air.

For most of my adult life, I believed that I could drop the extra weight I was carrying around by simply dieting for a little while. That may very well work in the short term, which is about as far as I ever got, but it won't cut it in the long term. To make it there, you need what the three examples above show: persistence.

With persistence, you can accomplish anything you set your mind to, whether it's making your first million or shedding almost 200 pounds of excess fat from your body. If you persist, you will not fail. You *cannot* fail. Failure becomes impossible with persistence. Sure, you may have temporary setbacks from time to time. I might even go so far as to say minor setbacks are to be expected. Persistence is what gets you past the setbacks.

According to the dictionary, the root of the word persistence comes from French and means "to take a stand" or to "stand firm." See how it works? If you stand firm in your resolution to do anything, weight-related or not, you'll continually monitor your progress and will know right away if you're moving off track to your final goal. If you move off track, realize it, and get back on.

Come with me. Let us persist.

October 23

I drink lots of water, between 64 and 128 ounces per day. I don't measure it, because I believe drinking is somewhat like eating – drink when you're thirsty, not because you have to consume some arbitrary amount of water every day to "maximize" the fat-shedding process. And yes, I've been told that if I'm thirsty, it's too late.

I don't want to get up every morning and subtract 150 from my base weight, then add 8 ounces to another base of 64 ounces for every 25 pounds over 150 I weigh, divided by the square root of the day of the month, just to know how much water some "expert" somewhere says I should drink. In like manner, I don't want to multiply my body weight by some arbitrary factor to calculate my caloric intake, or subtract my age from some other number to find my "optimal" exercise heart rate.

Call me a rebel, but life's too short to spend all my time counting things.

Don't get me wrong, if these things work for you, great. I believe in the "whatever it takes" philosophy. I just happen to believe "whatever it takes" ultimately boils down to being sensible about what I put into my body most of the time, instead of worrying about so many details.

October 24

Old habits die hard, but you know what I've found? They do die. And when they do, you don't miss them very much. For example, one of the biggest habits I once had was eating loads of sugary sweet food, like Oreos, Little Debbie snack cakes, and Ben and Jerry's ice cream. When I had the moment I refer to as finding my pain, I stopped eating sweets for several months.

My pain was strong enough that I didn't crave these foods at all for quite some time. About three or four weeks ago, I started having cravings for these foods. I allowed myself to give in, to see what would happen, and found that I don't care for the really sweet stuff at all now. The habit died, because I starved it to death.

Granted, I eat some sweet stuff now, like the occasional bowl of cereal or a blueberry muffin. Last night, I ate a few graham crackers. What's funny is that I went so long without eating anything sweet that semi-sweet foods now seem very sweet, and super-sweet foods are downright disgusting.

Robyn made fun of me last night, because I was telling her that eating things like a bowl of raisin nut bran or some graham crackers make my throat burn. There was a time when I could eat the better part of a bag of cookies in one sitting, but I doubt now that I could eat more than two or three. Killing an old habit has that effect. It removes the "need" from a certain food, and puts that food back into its proper place – something to be enjoyed, but sparingly.

One of the biggest helps to breaking a bad food habit is to simply pick up some new healthy habits. Try exercising every day and eating healthy food almost all the time. When you do that for a while then try to eat something unhealthy, your body reacts as though you've ingested poison.

Which, in a sense, I guess you have.

October 29

While Robyn and Danielle were having dinner yesterday, I drove down to Walmart to buy some accoutrements for my bike. I got a water bottle for long rides, and a taillight that is reflective in the day, and flashes at night. In addition to that, I bought a battery-powered, halogen headlight so oncoming traffic can see me puttering down the road (as though they could miss something as big as me). But, I do ride in the dark, so I figure I'll do whatever it takes to keep me from body-shaping the grill of an 18-wheeler.

I installed all the equipment on my bike last night, and took it for a test ride in the neighborhood. "Dork" is the closest word I can think of to describe how I must look, tooling along, headlight shining off the front end, taillight lighting up my ass in a red glow, and with a futuristic-looking water bottle sticking up from between my legs.

Riding this morning, I had my first interaction with motorists. A truckload of teen boys rode by and honked their horn at me. I smiled at them, because I knew they were impressed with my fancy setup. Sure enough, they passed me again, this time coming from the opposite direction. One of them leaned out the window as they went by and shouted, "Nice fuckin' bike!"

Nice fuckin' bike, indeed.

November 2000

280-275 pounds

November 3

Without warning this morning, suddenly it dawned on me that I weigh almost a hundred pounds less today than I did just a little over five months ago. The thought came over me in an instant, and I got as giddy as a schoolgirl when I realized how far I've already come.

There were days that seemed eternal, and I wondered if it would be worth all the time I was spending. Time crawled, and I'd have thoughts along the lines of, "I'll be eating the same way for the rest of my life, yuck." Through it all, though, I held on to one image – that of a fit and buff me. I'm not there yet, but I think I'm more than halfway. In retrospect, the five months seem to have passed in a flash. I feel like yesterday I was a blimp, and today I'm only a balloon. Seeing this, I realize that tomorrow I'll be there, right where I want to be.

You can join me if you like. It all starts with a decision.

November 14

We went to Gatlinburg again, just so I could do all the things I'd wanted to do back in May. On Friday, I went through the Ripley's Believe It or Not museum, rode the earthquake ride, went through Ripley's Haunted Adventure, through the World of Illusions, and to see a 3-D movie.

On Saturday, we rode the tram up the mountain to Ober Gatlinburg and back down. Afterwards, while Robyn and Danielle waited out front, I rode the Motion Theater ride, where the seats beat me senseless. I loved it, but Robyn and Danielle didn't care for the wait.

Saturday afternoon was my *coup de grace*. We went to Dollywood for the afternoon and I'm pleased to say that after ten years of not being able to, I took a ride on the Tennessee Tornado, a roller coaster. I liked it so much I rode twice, and would have ridden many more times had Robyn and Danielle not been getting so cold.

It's so nice being able to fit again.

November 27

I wore my 46-inch-waist pants to work today. I'd stopped wearing them because they were working some hell on my testicles, fitting fine in the waist but making it feel like someone had my genitals in a firm squeeze whenever I sat. A fine thing when I'm with my wife, perhaps, but not the sort of thing I want to deal with at the office.

In any case, they're now loose enough to put on and take off without even unbuttoning them, and they no longer make me worry about becoming sterile. My 48-inch-pants, which I put on yesterday, have become obscenely big on me. It would appear that I'm reshaping still, even though there's no significant weight coming off these days.

November 29

I wore some of my "fat" pants to work today, the ones with the 52-inch waist, because I still haven't thrown out all the old clothes. I drink a lot of water when I'm working, and inevitably pee a lot. On one such occasion, I zipped my pants and stepped over to the sink to wash my hands. I saw myself in the mirror, and something didn't look quite right, so I turned a little for a closer look. My left back pocket was on the side of my hip.

Why don't people *tell* me when I spend the day walking around looking like a freak?

November 30

There is a certain story told about an old carpenter who was ready to retire. His boss the contractor was sorry to see him retiring and asked him to build one last house as a personal favor because he was such a good carpenter. The carpenter agreed and began work on the house. After a while, thinking of the time he could be spending fishing instead of working, he slacked off and built a large portion of the house shoddily, using poor workmanship and inferior materials.

When he finished the house, he brought the contractor over for the final inspection. Standing on the front porch of the house, the contractor handed the keys to the house to the carpenter and said, "This house is my gift to you, for so many years of good service."

All too often we tend to treat our bodies the same way the old carpenter treated the house. We don't realize until the end, it seems, that we're building our bodies for ourselves, not some faceless stranger.

We use materials that are definitely inferior. In my case, it was Big Macs, Oreos, and Little Debbie. For you it may be different. Inferior materials create an inferior product, one that's morbidly obese, disease-prone, and ready for an early grave. We choose to sit on our butts, rather than work at building a house that we're proud to live in. Without some sort of realization in this building process, you end up with a shoddy house, surprised in the end that it's yours.

There is hope, however.

Your house can be repaired. Remodeling is not terribly difficult, because your house wants to be built properly – to be strong and healthy, ready to stand against the storms and termites life offers. All you have to do is supply the proper materials and good craftsmanship.

December 2000

274 – 270 *pounds*

December 3

During my exercise this morning, I noticed something that made me happy. My right leg, the weaker one, doesn't really seem to have a knee problem any more. The ankle has been the worst part, but the knee pained me from time to time, particularly going up and down stairs. In any case, I realized that not only has it not bothered me in over a month, I'm able to crouch lower both in kickboxing and in the walking videos I do.

When I came out of the exercise room I decided to test my ankle – which still hurts if I jog too much – on the stairs. For the last several years I've walked down the stairs funny, left leg down a stair and then the right leg following to the same riser, like a small child. This was due to the aforementioned knee. On the occasions when I tried to walk down the stairs in a normal manner, my right leg would slam loudly into the lower stair, because it would hit heel-first rather than toe-first. I sounded like some sort of Frankenstein monster hobbling my way down to a dungeon.

In my test this morning, I'm pleased to say that I can now walk down the stairs like a normal person. I just have to break out of the habit of my former, odd gait now.

December 7

All too often we tend to feel the need to pass responsibility for our decisions and actions off onto someone else, particularly with regards to our weight. We become victims – of time, other people, and food, to name a few – in order to shun our responsibilities. The victim mentality will keep you obese, right up until the fat squeezes your heart in a final death grip or the granules of sugar in your blood destroy everything inside you. Mark my words, it *will* win unless you grab the proverbial bull by the horns and take responsibility for yourself.

An acquaintance looked a little down the week before last, and I asked him if everything was all right. He told me that one of his friends dropped dead of a heart attack suddenly during the previous weekend. This friend was distraught, because the dead man was apparently in good shape and was pretty young. I suspect this acquaintance saw a glimpse of his own mortality and it frightened him because he's overweight and doesn't exercise.

"I guess I'll be eating salads from now on," he said to me.

The next morning we were on the phone, and he mentioned he'd been eating a Croissan'wich and some hash rounds from Burger King. Being the annoying fat-person-who's-dropped-a-lot-of-weight that I am (quite possibly worse than an ex-smoker, even), I said, "What about the salad you were going to eat?"

His response? He "didn't have time" to buy some healthy food. It appears he still hasn't had time, because he's invited me to lunch at a local grease joint several times over the last week.

Don't turn yourself into a victim of time, of circumstance, of *anything*. Take responsibility for yourself. I spent a great deal of my life putting that responsibility off on other people and things, until I finally woke up and took control. If you're a victim, you're letting someone or something else run your life, and that's no life at all.

December 9

Recently I was at a large sit-down lunch, and it came to light as the food was delivered that I hadn't ordered anything.

"Didn't you know? Fred's on a diet!" someone offered.

Nothing annoys me quite as much as when a skinny person does something like this. It's like they don't realize how it makes us fatties feel. Makes *me* feel, anyway. Perhaps I'm just sensitive, who knows?

December 20

This morning when I walk-jogged it was 11 degrees out. Eleven. Degrees.

The hair in my nose froze, or at least it felt like it. And there was one brief time when I wiped at my nose and thought it was going to snap off, fall to the sidewalk, and shatter into a spray of glistening pink crystals, but it didn't.

December 22

Given the time of year, and the fact that I'm 100 pounds lighter, I'd like to take this opportunity to reflect on the new things in my life. I've done this before, so some of it may be familiar, but here goes:

- My waist is about ten inches smaller.
- I weigh just a little more than I did in 1990 when I graduated college.
- I can run again.
- Not only can I run, I can run for more than a mile in my morning exercise.
- Sex is more pleasurable.
- My face looks human.
- I can go up several flights of stairs without breathing hard.
- I can do pushups.
- My legs and ankles no longer ache.
- I last longer during sex.
- My penis is larger because the fat around it is receding.
- I am not a diabetic.
- I don't get yeast infections or boils from having high blood sugar.
- I'm medicine-free.
- My blood pressure is down.
- I haven't gotten sick since I started this process.
- My wife and daughter can both reach around me now, easily.
- I can exercise for an hour or more without feeling any pain.
- I fit in roller coaster seats.
- I'm one size away from the normal man's store.
- My shirt size has dropped 3 X's.
- My neck is several inches smaller.
- I can walk all day in Gatlinburg, *after* walking 3 miles in the morning.

- My wedding ring falls off now.
- I rarely take naps.
- I don't snore unless I'm on my back.
- I don't have heartburn.
- I don't have apnea.
- I sleep the night through.
- I feel better than I can remember.
- I'm no longer embarrassed to go in public.
- I'm not ashamed to run into people from my thinner past.
- I can ride a bike again.
- I'll be riding a scooter soon.
- I have more energy than ever before.
- I can cut my own toenails.
- I fit in theater seats.
- I fit in booths at restaurants.
- I don't need the jumbo smock when I get my hair cut.
- My thighs don't chafe.
- I can wear pullovers without being ashamed of my boobs.
- I don't mind having my picture taken any more.
- My self-esteem is much higher.
- I'm more flexible and agile.
- I love myself again.

December 26

My running distance is gradually increasing – I ran 1.5 miles today. It's nice, because I stay a little sore all the time now. When I started this whole weight-dropping thing, I stayed sore all the time and I liked it because it made me feel as though I were accomplishing something. Until I started pushing myself, I'd stopped being sore, and I think I may not have been exercising hard enough.

December 29

Yesterday I received in the mail two pairs of jeans I ordered off the web. Both pairs of pants are 44 inches in the waist, and look great, but there's a small problem.

They're too big.

However, it's nice to have pants where the crotch is in the crotch, instead of around my knees. It's amazing to me that I continue to shrink somewhat significantly while my weight continues to move down so slowly. I think maybe I need to just be quiet and not so concerned with a number on a scale and be more concerned with the knowledge that I've dropped about 10 inches off my waist. Or care more about the fact that I run more than a mile a day, every day. Or even that I can fit in restaurant booths and amusement park rides whenever I want to.

Have I mentioned that the normal men's store waist sizes go up to 42? I'm almost there, size-wise.

January 2001

269 – 260 pounds

January 1

A new year is upon us, and I enter it weighing a mere 9.5 pounds more than I did when I graduated from college in December of 1990. I now weigh 269 pounds.

With each New Year's Day come the inevitable resolutions people make. Did you make any this year? I didn't. I used to, but then I realized I never really kept them because I didn't think about them until the *next* new year had rolled in.

Who needs resolutions? Just *do* it.

January 3

Almost daily I am reminded of how much most people take for granted. For example, I was talking today with a friend about an annual picnic that will be coming up in July, sponsored by my company's largest customer. For the last few years, I've avoided this picnic because I was embarrassed to seen by so many people at once.

The last two or three times I went this particular friend went too, and brought a pontoon boat each time. He used the boat to take people tubing on the Tennessee River, which was always a big hit. Each time, I rode on the boat with him, but I never rode the inner tube, which seemed to bother my friend. He assumed it was because I didn't trust him behind the wheel of his boat.

Just today, he and I were talking about this picnic again and I pointed out that I have every intention of going, just to show off my new body. He asked once again if I would ride the inner tube this year. I said that indeed I would, and went on to explain to him just why I hadn't done it before. It's simple, really. I was afraid I wouldn't be able to climb out of the water and into the boat. I'd seen plenty of skinny people have trouble doing this, to the point of almost having to be lifted up, and I knew there was no way in hell I could do it on my own, not weighing in at close to 400 pounds.

The look of surprise on his face was almost comical, and I realized the thought had never crossed his mind. He assumed that most everyone would have about the same level of difficulty getting out of the water, because he took it for granted. I get this a lot, especially when I'm telling people things like, "I'm one size away from the normal man's store!" excitedly.

Someone who's never shopped for super-sized clothes doesn't understand how good that feels. Or how it feels to sit in a theater seat without being squeezed painfully between the arms of the seat. The same goes for airplane seats. I always flew first class, not because I'm a snob but because I couldn't fit comfortably in the coach seats.

The list could go on forever. We take so many things for granted that we lose sight of the daily struggles so many people around us have. As big as I was, there were things I took for granted that others cannot do because of their size.

I could walk. I could sit in a single chair. I could sleep lying down, instead of sitting up so my own weight didn't smother me.

That list could go on forever, too. Take some time and think about all the things you take for granted that others don't. Then think about all the things other people take for granted that make you struggle. It's sobering.

January 6

I played racquetball Thursday for the first time in years. I won two games and lost three. That's okay, though, because I got an incredible workout: 75 minutes with my heart rate averaging 153 beats per minute. Not too shabby, considering when I walk-jog my heart rate averages 120-130 during the 45 or so minutes I'm out doing that.

Damn, I'm sore today. Especially my ass.

January 8

My home gym weight set has been calling to me again. "Fred," it whispers, "come play with me. Lift my weights and make yourself buff."

I'm cracking, and I'm about to give in.

January 11

My skin, particularly that on my abdomen, is getting grossly loose. Last night while laying in bed talking to my wife, I casually reached down and grabbed the bottom part of my abdomen in one hand, and the part a couple of inches above my belly button in the other, and was able to bring the sections together, creating a fold that was about 2.5 inches deep. Gross.

January 15

I lifted weights today for the first time. I'm a total wimp. My arms cannot lift *nearly* the weight I thought they could. So much for feeling like a big stud when I'm walking around the house, I suppose.

I feel like I haven't gotten any exercise at all. My legs are begging me to go for a walk-jog, or for a walk at the very least. They're crying, "Fred, what's up? Why you didn't exercise us today? Don't you still love us?"

I'm going for a walk, damn it, so I don't go crazy.

January 17

Today is day two of my weight training, and I was going to work out my lower body, but I got a rude awakening when I climbed onto the home gym. Apparently, three months of running (literally) around with a body that's almost 300 pounds does some major work to the legs, and the paltry 150 pounds on the machine wasn't nearly enough to work my stone-cut and super-buff legs to exhaustion. So I did the next best thing.

I did abdominal work and went for a nice walk-jog.

It's funny really, when you think about it. My original plan was to drop a chunk of weight, then use weight training to bulk up my shoulders, arms, and pectorals (not that my man-boobs need to be any bigger) in order to end up with an overall classic male shape: wide at the shoulders, narrow at the waist and hips. You know what I mean.

Apparently I didn't need to outthink myself in the middle of the game.

January 20

It's official. My two-week-old 42-inch-waist normal-sized pants are loose. I noticed yesterday that they were sagging dangerously low on my butt, to the point of exposing a good inch of crack. Fortunately, I was also wearing a low-hanging shirt. As it stands, I'm sitting here wearing a pair of 40-inch pants, and they feel just right.

January 29

Today's weigh-in puts me exactly 1.5 pounds above what I weighed when I graduated from college in December of 1990. What this means is that in eight months, I've mostly undone the ill effects of almost ten years of eating poorly and sitting on my ever widening behind.

Finding your pain is the defining moment when something happens, or when you discover something, that makes *not* changing yourself an impossible thing. For me, it was seeing a diabetic man have to have one of his legs amputated simply because he wasn't taking control of his life, something that I myself wasn't doing. As I watched this drama unfold, I was stuffing a Little Debbie strawberry roll into my fat face, and while the man wailed and cried about his loss, I had my moment of epiphany. That was eight months ago, and my life has changed dramatically since that time.

For one, I'm no longer a diabetic. No more pills; no more elevated blood sugar. I'm 110 pounds lighter, and I'd venture to say I'm in the best shape of my adult life, if not my whole life. I found my pain.

When I saw what that man was going through, I realized he was where I was going to be in just a few years. My future lay in my hands, ready for me to take hold and shape. Staying the way I was became an impossible task, because the thought of losing limbs was so painful to me. The rest is history.

Have you found your pain?

January 30

When I started the transformation from chunk to hunk, I knew there were going to be three stages. First, I had to get my eating under control. Then, my plan was to start weight training. I've done both of those, and though it's a little more premature than I originally planned, I feel the time is ripe to begin what I fondly think of as stage three of my transformation.

Yesterday, I quit smoking. I put the cigarettes down, and I won't be picking them back up. Common knowledge says that any time a person quits smoking, that person will gain weight because they replace the bad habit of smoking with the bad habit of overeating.

I think common knowledge needs to take a step back and learn that all things are possible if you believe in yourself.

January 31

Far too long I used excuses – large frame, denial, bad genes – for weighing almost 400 pounds. The simple truth was this: I weighed almost 400 pounds because I was an eating machine. Food was the center of my life. I was in a vicious cycle, because I hated how fat I was and that hatred just made me eat more. I was digging my grave with a fork and a spoon until I got my wakeup call and found that it was, in fact, possible to love myself enough to take charge of my life.

Life is all about choices. You can choose wisely, or you can choose poorly. How will you choose? Don't get me wrong, no one's perfect, and we all make our share of poor choices when it comes to eating or exercise. Aim for a *tendency* to make wise choices, not perfection. When your tendency is to choose wisely, there's no need to beat yourself up over an individual poor choice. For example, I had a big bowl of popcorn a couple of days ago with a half-stick of butter and a good bit of Parmesan cheese. Was it a wise choice for a snack? Probably not, but my tendency over that day and even over the whole week was to make wise choices, and I'll not feel bad for making one poor choice.

February 2001

259 – 251 *pounds*

February 2

Are you perfect?

I'm not, either. Why then do we mentally abuse ourselves for our imperfections? I cannot speak for any of you reading this right now, but I can speak for myself, and the abuse I once heaped upon my own head. Every time I made the decision to "lose weight," I'd be "good" for a few days, but I'd invariably slip, due possibly to some unforeseen event or stress, and my intentions were suddenly shot to hell.

I'd make declarations that I was just destined to be fat and that was that. I'd call Domino's and order a large pizza and consume it by myself, my eyes on the television so I didn't have to think about what I was doing to myself. I'd failed, you see, in my own eyes, because I wasn't "perfect," and therefore unworthy of my ultimate goal.

It might be argued that I strove for perfection when I started down the path I'm on now because I went several months without eating sugar, and because I made consistently healthful choices when it came time to put food in my mouth. That wasn't perfection, though, that was fear. Death and dismemberment were powerful motivators then, but my motivation has changed now, mostly because I'm not in any danger of either.

Somewhere over the last three or four months, eating right and exercising ceased being "something I'm doing" and became a permanent part of my life. Rather than being motivated by my initial fear, I'm motivated by just how *good* I feel now.

I want to talk about perfection, because I think it's a leading cause of why so many people fail to achieve their dreams. Let me just be blunt:

perfection is not going to work. There's something better than perfection, anyway, something that guarantees success. If you do this, you will succeed, whether it's in dropping excess weight, getting physically fit, or even making your first million. What is it? Improvement.

Rather than aiming for being perfect, just aim to be little bit better today than you were yesterday. You won't fail if you're not perfect, you'll fail if you're not committed to improving yourself slightly each day. Did you eat more than your body needs today? That's fine, stop dwelling on the past. Eat a little less tomorrow. It really is that simple. Did you skip exercising, perhaps? Again, it is not the end of the world. Just make sure you make a little progress tomorrow. That progress might be walking to the end of the street and back, or it might be running 10 miles. We're all different.

I don't want to be perfect. I just want to be a little better each day, and it's working.

February 5

I now weigh less than I did when I graduated from college in 1990.

When I decided last Monday to stop smoking, I took a little time to rework my mental image of myself. Instead of looking at myself as a smoker who's quitting, I made the decision that I'm simply a non-smoker.

There's a subtle difference there, believe it or not.

A smoker (or a fat person) who's "trying to quit" ("trying to lose weight") is focusing on deprivation, in a sense, because of all the connotations society has put on making this sort of change. By redefining my view of myself into someone who doesn't smoke, there's no desire at all to light up a cigarette, because lighting one up is no longer part of Fred.

Since I'm not a smoker who's attempting to quit, but a non-smoker, how can I possibly want to smoke? Yes, I really *do* think it's that simple.

February 8

I went to see my accountant today because there's a bit of tax work he needs to do for me. I walked through the door to his office to find him bent over his assistant at her computer, helping her with something on the screen. They both looked up at me.

And looked, and looked. I could almost see the "something's different with Fred" wheels turning in their heads. It's been, after all, almost a year since I've seen them.

Finally, they decided I looked younger. I said, "I get younger every day!" and that was that.

February 9

I spent a large number of years planning to change things either "tomorrow" or "Monday," depending on the time of day or day of the week. Merely planning to lose weight never got me too far. In fact, one could easily argue that I *planned* my way up to almost 400 pounds. The road to hell is, after all, paved with good intentions.

Obviously, you have to have a plan in order to accomplish something of great magnitude, and I don't mean to suggest that one should never make plans. I do have a plan: to be fit and healthy by July of this year, and to enjoy the ride along the way. This plan is written down, and it covers the things I need to do to make sure I accomplish what I set out to do. It's specific, not some nebulous idea waiting to be put off or forgotten. You need a plan like that. It's a roadmap to success; it is a goal to be achieved. That use of the word "plan" is the transitive sense, meaning, "to design; to devise or project the realization of."

The version of the word "plan" that's the killer is the *in*transitive form, which means "to have in mind; to intend." Used in the sentence, "I intend to change, but I'm not going to because I'm not willing to take any immediate action toward achieving my goal."

Don't let your road through life be simply paved with good intentions. Set your mind to accomplish great things, write down a plan for achieving them, and make it happen.

You'll never be the same.

February 10

I have a strange physical situation. Though I'm still very fat, over the last week or so I've noticed bulges in all the right places on my stomach. They're in the magic spots where every man wants them, and I can only come to one conclusion.

I think I have a baby six-pack hiding under the fat.

February 12

Today a friend told me that another of his friends, who I'd run into last week, asked him if I had cancer. I laughed. Not, of course, at the thought of having cancer, but that someone might think I did just because I'm so much smaller now.

Perhaps this is why those skinny folks don't ever say, "Are you losing weight?"

They're afraid you're dying.

February 15

There are a great number of people in this world looking for the answer to dropping weight. I see them regularly online, asking for plans of what to eat, how to eat, when to eat.

Should I try high carbohydrate and low protein? Should I try high protein and low carbohydrate? How many calories should I eat each day? Should I exercise? How much? How often?

Never fear, I'm here to answer.

Humankind never had a problem with obesity until recently. We've started to rely far too much on processed foods, and we don't have anywhere near the physical activity our forefathers did. We sit on our butts watching television and eating our candy and chips then wonder why we puff up like marshmallows. I read a magazine article just yesterday about obese children. The average child today plays outside for seventeen minutes a day. Seventeen minutes! It's no wonder we're a fat nation.

Here's the answer, nice and simple: Think about what you put into your mouth. Before you pop the lid off the ice cream, ask yourself a question – will this food help me or harm me? Maximize the helpful foods and minimize the harmful ones.

Get off the couch. Move. Play like a child again (like when *you* were a child, not like today's kids). You don't need a pill, and you don't need any kind of surgery. No fad diets, no cabbage soup, no deprivation. It works; I give you my word as someone who's done it. The biggest problem we have today is that we eat too many harmful (read: convenience) foods and don't move our bodies enough.

February 16

I contend that one can eat whatever he wants and still drop weight. There's a caveat to that, though, it's not a magic bullet for success. Obviously, there's a moderation issue; you cannot eat a couple of pounds of butter a day and reasonably expect to get good health out of it. There's another part to this picture, however, and it lies in your head.

If you work on the mental side of eating, you can modify your thought processes so the unhealthy things don't appeal to you. Think of it in the same terms as "finding your pain," only with what you eat.

For example, I saw someone in a local grocery store yesterday buying his lunch: a Styrofoam plate loaded with barbecue-sauce-coated slices of greasy Polish sausage and deep-fried squash and potatoes. I only know what the squash and potatoes were because I heard him order them. The thick layer of breading covering them made them unrecognizable. The meal also came with a large white roll and a Coke. To round it all out, this person had picked up a box of cookies for dessert.

This is the sort of meal I once ate almost daily.

Do you like the smell of hot grease? I don't. It grosses me out, and just smelling it reminds me of the time I saw a doctor pull a length of plaque out of a man's artery. That greasy smell was just rolling out of the Styrofoam container in the man's hand.

What about the feel of grease all around your mouth, on your hands, and coating your tongue? Do you like that? Do you enjoy leaving greasy skid marks on whatever you touch? What about the effect of the grease on your feces? Do you enjoy sluggish bowel movements?

Have you ever tried to exercise after eating something really unhealthy, like fried foods? How did you feel? Did you exercise better or worse than normal? Do you like the bloated and heavy feeling that comes with foods like that?

How about drinking a cup of nice warm oil? Ever done that? Would you like to? Imagine it sliding down your throat, all thick and slimy, the little crunchies of fried breading crushing between your teeth. How about letting that oil firm up into something like Crisco, then pulling a sheet of the hardened fat off and eating it? Think about how it would make your teeth feel, think about it coating your tongue and turning it white.

The sausage, squash, and potatoes await you. Go ahead, you can have all you want.

February 21

It's official. My 42-inch pants are far too big now, my 40-inch pants fit comfortably loosely, and I can now wear the 38-inchers around the house. They're a tad tighter than I'd want to sit in at a desk all day, but great for lounging on the couch, as I'm wont to do.

February 24

Dear King Size Direct,

I am in receipt of your latest catalog, which arrived in my mailbox today, presumably because my single purchase from your website last year put me on your mailing list. While your clothes appear to be quite nice (and I must point out you have some very handsome models, though I wonder why none of them are fat), they're no longer for me. Shortly after I ordered those XXXXXL shirts from you last year, I took charge of my life and dropped over 100 pounds.

As a result, I am merely a large man, and no longer "king sized" by any stretch of the imagination. I no longer have any need to receive your advertising or catalogs. Please consider this letter my request for you to remove me from your mailing list. I have included the back page from your catalog so you can find the reference information necessary to remove me.

Thank you for your prompt attention in this matter.

Sincerely,
Fred Anderson

February 26

Yesterday was gorgeous here, about 70 degrees and mostly clear with only a few high fluffy clouds. Since I'm still not 100% comfortable with the thought of riding in traffic (I still wobble on occasion, lacking practice), I loaded the bike into the Jeep and went to my daughter's school, where they have a quarter-mile track. I was enjoying myself immensely, my hair flying and a big grin on my face, out in public for the first time in over a decade wearing a t-shirt.

Ultimately I rode around the track 28 times, giving me a total of 7 miles, which was a nice ride. I wasn't aiming for more cardio (I'd already run that morning), but I got some because I really like to push it when I'm on the bike. My treks on the big circle were grand, but there was a bad moment right in the middle.

A mother showed up with her two kids.

Mom and the daughter were walking, and the son was on his bike. He looked to be about seven. They came onto the track just after I passed the sidewalk they were on, going the opposite direction I was. The boy took off in the lead, pumping his legs as fast as he could. He rounded the end furthest from me and looked up at me.

And got a panicky gleam in his eyes. I could see the wheels turning inside his head. *Oh shit,* they said, *this guy's moving fast for such a fat guy. I need to stay out of his way!* I watched him come around the track toward me, he on the inside and me on the outside, and his eyes never left me once.

I knew what was coming, because I preach this principle.

About 50 feet from me, he did a big arcing swerve directly into my path. I had to stand up on the brakes and skid to a stop to keep from hitting him. He grinned and swerved back into his lane and past me. His mother yelled at him from the other side of the track.

I've said it once, and I'll say it again: you go toward whatever you focus on.

If you whine and complain and moan about how hard it is to drop weight, guess what? For you, it'll be hard. If you focus on how you've always been fat, you'll probably stay fat, or even get fatter. If you think about how much you hate exercise because it's so hard, it's going to stay hard.

I choose focus on being a fit and healthy man, and my mind's taking me right to that. When I'm asked what my plan is, I say this: "I live like the man I want to be."

And I'm becoming that man. When I look in the mirror, I see the Fred who'll be here for good in just a few months, not the Fred who's here right now, and definitely not the one from a few months back. When it's time to eat, I eat like the man who's on his way, not the man who's here currently. When I get up to exercise, I work out like that man, not this one.

Live it, and become it.

February 28

I fear that I may have been optimistic in my original calculations of fourteen months to drop all my weight. I hate being wrong. With about 66 pounds to go to 185 (my floating goal) and five months until the end of July, that would mean I need to drop about 13 pounds a month, or roughly 3 pounds a week from now until then. Looking at my performance over the last few months, I don't anticipate that happening.

Don't get me wrong, I could *make* it happen, but the point is to live like the man I want to be, not to drop a certain number of pounds by a certain date. To guarantee 3 pounds a week, I could cut out some of my food or increase my exercise, but then I wouldn't feel as though I were living the way I wanted to.

I think I'll be close, probably within 10 or 15 pounds (depending, of course, on several factors), and that's just fine with me. If it takes me an extra month, or even two, I'll not consider myself a failure. Missing a goal does not make one a failure.

Giving up does.

March 2001

250 – 243 pounds

March 2

I had my first bicycle wreck today. In my office. Fortunately the wall, the table, and I are all doing well, and I have learned a valuable lesson about showing off.

Mostly.

⁂

I was in Walmart today getting some contact lenses (my face is not bloated and fat now, and no longer wants to hide behind fat man glasses) when the subject of weight loss came up. The optician, it turns out, is my age and has dropped 60 pounds himself. He told me he put the weight on by too much partying in his youth and too many trips to the fast food places after late-night drinking at bars. Know what he told me when I asked him what he'd done to transform himself?

He changed his beliefs about food.

I kid you not, those are his words, not mine. He said he decided eating garbage all the time just wasn't worth the extra fat and associated problems (apnea, snoring, and heartburn were a few of the things he mentioned) that came with it. So, he made a decision to stop eating processed foods and to stick with natural foods. As simple as that, he's a new man.

March 4

Lying in bed Thursday night and talking with my wife, I made the comment in passing that one day I'd love to start running at the bottom of our driveway and run all the way to the end of the street without stopping, a total distance of six-tenths of a mile.

Currently, I interval train when I run. I call it walk-jogging, because I alternate walking and jogging. Normally, I walk for the first two tenths of a mile or so, to warm up my legs, then run until I feel like stopping. Most days this is at the end of the street, but on occasion I don't make it that far.

Friday morning, thinking of the comment I'd made the previous night, I decided the present was a good time to start working on my dream of running from my driveway to the end of the street nonstop. So, instead of walking to the point where I normally do, I started running about a tenth of a mile sooner. I made it to the end of the street without stopping. As a matter of fact, I pushed myself a little harder all the way through my run, and ran 2.7 miles altogether, a new personal record.

Yesterday, I started running a little closer to my driveway, and again made it to the end of my street without stopping. I ran a total of 2.6 miles. Not a record, but very close.

I woke up this morning at about 3:50, and it was pouring rain. The wind was blowing loudly, and lightning was flashing.

Great, I thought, *this is just what I need.*

I stayed in bed until about 4:30, until I could no longer hear any rain, then rolled out and got dressed. I walked out of the garage, and stopped for a second with my eyes closed. In my mind's eye, I saw the new Fred start running at the end of the driveway, and not stop at all until he got to the end of the street. He felt good, and he looked good, and he didn't falter during that six-tenths of a mile.

I opened my eyes, walked to the bottom of the driveway, and hit the play button on my Walkman. I took a deep breath and started running. About four tenths of a mile down the road, my legs whined at me a little – *hey, Fred, c'mon, it's time to stop, isn't it?* – but I ignored them. They didn't hurt, but they were ready to take it easy. The Fred I saw in my head was still going strong, so I kept running and sure enough, they stopped whining just a few seconds later.

I ran from my driveway to the end of the street. And I kept going. All in all, I ran about 1.3 miles before I stopped to walk for a tenth of a mile. Then I was off again, running like a fool through a second subdivision and back home.

I won't lie, I'm a little stiff now, and I may very well be sore tomorrow. That's fine; it's a weightlifting and bike day. There's something more important than that that I want to impress upon you.

Visualization works. Get the image in your head, believe in yourself, and make your dream come true. See yourself succeeding in your mind's eye, and then succeed.

March 5

When talking about physical transformations, one hears the word "motivation" a lot. Generally people want to know how I stay motivated to keep eating healthy, and dropping weight. I wish I had a good answer, but the fact of the matter is I'm no longer motivated. Listen closely: I didn't say anything about going back to the man I used to be. I said I wasn't motivated. There's a big difference.

Let me ask a question, and I'd like for you to think about it for a minute. Are you motivated to brush your teeth each morning? No, it's just something you do. In the same way, choosing healthy foods most of the time and exercising each day are just something I do now. There's no motivation involved at all. And that's what makes it so easy.

March 8

If your food has *quality*, you don't need to worry so much about *quantity*.

For example, a Big Mac from McDonald's (one of the old Fred's favorites) has about 600 calories. Here are a few other things with about 600 calories: a little more than two pounds of shrimp; three 8-ounce chicken breasts; 30 cups of bagged salad; 8.5 apples; 12 cups of puffed wheat; almost a half gallon of skim milk; six cups of cooked oatmeal; 12 slices of whole wheat bread.

See my point? I don't worry about quantities because 98% of what I eat comes from quality foods. I don't know about you, but I'd be hard pressed to eat any of the quantities of food above. A Big Mac, should I ever desire one, would be easy to eat because it's so small. Matter of fact, I used to eat a couple of fish sandwiches and one or two super-sized fries *in addition* to a Big Mac when I went to McDonald's.

I refer to this technique as choosing foods with a good "bang for the buck."

March 11

We fat people are a desperate bunch. We buy our books and read them, we try our fad diets, we pop our pills, and we visit the bariatric surgeons as a last resort. We talk about making a "lifestyle change," going on a diet, we have our support groups, and we still have over a 90% failure rate (note: bariatric surgery only fails a third of the time). Why is that? We look to the external for a solution to our weight problems, when the real solution – the permanent solution – is internal. I suggest instead of making a "lifestyle change" you consider making a "mindstyle change." If you change the way you think about eating, your body will take care of itself, I promise.

As a simple example, think for a minute what food means to you. Is it a comfort thing? A taste thing? An emotional thing? If you changed your core beliefs about food, what would happen?

Suppose you modified your view of food so that you see it as fuel – something necessary to sustain your life rather than something to be obsessed over, coveted, and longed-for? What then? Would that change what you put into your body? Which would your automobile rather have, the cheapest gas with all the additives or some super high-octane 100% pure premium gas? I'll take the premium fuel, please. Leave the crappy gas for the people who want their car to break down before it even has 40,000 miles on it.

Changing a belief is simple. Change the mind, and the body will change to follow.

March 13

Americans spend *thirty-three billion dollars* each year on the diet industry, and according to the latest (December 2000) statistics I could find, some 61% of American adults are still overweight. Wake up, America, it's not working.

As always, I have some comments. I consider myself something of an expert on being fat, since I spent all of my life at least a little fat, and the last ten years being super-fat. I know fat, and I know *why* I was fat. While there were several reasons, there was one main reason, and that is that I was simply lazy. *Lazy*. I didn't take the time to provide proper nutrition for myself; rather I ate fast food and junk food all the time because they were convenient and, let's face it, they tasted pretty good. I took the easy way out. I was not alone – Americans are eating, on average, 148 calories more per day than we did 20 years ago.

Not only was I lazy when choosing what to eat, I was lazy in a very physical sense. I write software for a living, which means I basically spend my day sitting on my butt at a computer. At home I was no different, still sitting and looking at one thing or another. All the things we've invented to make our lives easier have come back to haunt us with a particular ferocity.

Both of my grandfathers worked with their hands. Grandpa Fred was a farmer, and Grandpa Walter was a construction man. They didn't have computers, or televisions, or fancy cars. Those things (computers excluded) were luxuries. They didn't have to exercise because exercise was a part of their lives. They were also fit and healthy.

"Eat less and move more" is a nice formula, and I've been known to use it when someone I know walks up ands asks me the "secret" to dropping 125 pounds (that's my laziness showing back up). Saying that is a lot easier than going through all the different mental techniques I use, and it saves me the funny looks I get when I point to my head and say, "I changed this, and my body changed itself."

Eating less and moving more definitely work, because if you exclude all the things I say about the mental side, physically that's really what I've done to drop this weight. I consume many calories less (though I actually eat *more* food) than I did, and I move much more (at least for 45-90 minutes a day, now. I sit on my butt like always the rest of the day). If that's all you are looking for, the "secret to losing weight," then you've found it.

If, however, you're interested in looking deeper, looking beneath the platitudes, keep reading. Fix your mind, and watch your body fix itself.

March 19

Last May 28, I was presented with a choice that required a decision to be made. I had just thrown away my Little Debbie Banana Twins and Strawberry Roll because of that whole rotting foot thing on television, and I stood at the cusp of a life-changing moment. The key to how far I've come since that day was *not* seeing the image of the blackened toes on my TV, it was the decision I made to hold myself to a higher standard from that point forward.

Throwing the Little Debbie cake away was mostly involuntary, brought on by a horrifying and disgusting image. The doctor pointing out that the man was having the amputation due to his own poor decisions magnified the hurt. What I'm talking about here is the decision I made shortly after that instant, not the visceral reaction I had.

That decision brought me to where I am today. When I made that decision to regain my health, I immediately changed the path I was traveling, and resolved to live my life in a whole new way. I haven't looked back, and I don't plan to anytime soon.

When you make a decision, and thereby choose the path you're going to follow, there's one step that gives that decision some massive power, and that's taking immediate action. Suppose you decide to reclaim your life and control of what you're eating. Do something toward realizing your decision right away.

Not tomorrow. Not next week. Not next month. *Now.*

The biggest thing that holds people back is the ease with which a decision can be made, and then procrastinated upon. I spent ten years planning to do something about my health and weight at two different times: "tomorrow" or "Monday." Neither ever came. When I made the decision for the last time last May, I took immediate action. I threw away not only the Little Debbie cakes I was eating, but also all the junk food in the house that was designated as mine.

Don't make a life-changing decision without taking some action right away. Taking this action not only demonstrates the incredible power you have over your own destiny, it increases that power, because when you take the first action, no matter how simple, you're empowered to take a second and a third. The actions build upon themselves and before you know it, you're almost to the point that you once dreamed about. Trust me, I know.

March 22

I have a tendency to be anal about things, and I'd become anal about a couple of things in my life over the last couple of months. I became the kind of man I didn't want to be, with regards to food. Anal. Obsessive. Scared, almost at the thought of having something really unhealthy.

I haven't been out to eat since early January and even then I had a no-dressing salad, a plain potato, and boiled shrimp because I was put off that everything else on the menu appeared to be butter-broiled or fried. In my efforts to become the man of my dreams, I became the man of my nightmares. When I started, we'd eat out on Friday nights, and I'd have Taco Bell, or Arby's, or pizza, and I wouldn't think twice. I ate that way through over 100 pounds of fat Fred, and I didn't look back.

That is the man I want to be – the fit and healthy one who leads a balanced life, food-wise – not some freakish person who stops eating out because "nothing's healthy." It's all about keeping things in balance and perspective, and with food I lost that perspective. In my desire to transform, I obsessed over the same thing I spent my life obsessing over, but in a 180-degree manner.

No more. I know what's healthy, and I will continue to eat healthy foods. I'm eating out this Friday, however, and I'll not fret a bit if I eat something not so healthy. Such is life.

The one other place in my life where I feel I got unbalanced is with regards to exercise. Somehow, I have allowed myself to slide into the mindset that I have to exercise every morning at about 4 am, and that the world might very well end should I ever not do that one day.

I realized last night that in fact, the world would *not* end. Hell, it wouldn't even blink. So, to prove my point, when I woke up this morning at 4, I rolled back over and went to sleep until almost 5:30. I lifted weights after work and nothing bad happened at all.

Sometimes, I'm just a freak.

These points do, however, lead somewhere. I'm following a master plan, right now, one that's guaranteed me success in my transformation. There are several steps involved in this plan, but I'll promise that if you try it, you'll see that it works: make a decision. Take immediate action. Monitor your progress. If you don't like your results change your plan of attack and do it again. What could possibly be simpler?

March 26

On June 8, 2000, I wrote the following:

"I want to lose 120 pounds of body fat. I want to stop taking pills for diabetes. I want my blood sugar to be 100% NORMAL. I want to be able to play outside like a kid, and to fit into the amusement park rides I once loved. I want to be small enough to be easily straddled during sex. I want to be able to walk outside in the summertime and not sweat, and I want to be able to walk upstairs without limping and panting for breath. I want to look normal again."

Since I wrote that, I'm well over 100 pounds lighter. I no longer take pills for diabetes, and my blood sugar is 100% normal. Yesterday I took a nice fast bike ride like a kid, and today I spent almost a half hour playing Frisbee with some friends. I rode amusement park rides easily back in November, and can fit on any ride there is now. The sex is fine, too. We haven't had another summer since the last one, but I'm betting with the amount of time I spend complaining about how cold I am, over-sweating is not going to be an issue. I can run up and down the stairs, without limping and without my breath speeding up in the slightest. I look normal again.

Get a vision. Write it down. Make it happen.

March 28

I played Frisbee for about a half hour on Monday. Truly, I loved the freedom of running and jumping like a kid (well, like a kid in my head, anyway). I loved it so much that despite the tiny bit of soreness in my left bicep (my throwing arm), I went out yesterday afternoon after work and played Frisbee again. Played for almost 90 minutes, in fact.

I may play like a kid, but I sure hurt like an old man. As I write, the pain is pulsing across my shoulders and down both arms, all through my chest and abdomen, from my butt to my neck, and my left leg is throbbing like a rotting tooth. But, being able to play like that was worth every bit of it. Every little bit.

I wore my 38-inch pants to work today, because they fit comfortably now. I'm on the last hole of my newest belt, and there's still a bit of play in it.

❧

When I started my company with my partners, we made a 5-year-business plan. This plan is a roadmap for where my partners and I want to take our company, and we're following it pretty closely. It's our vision for the corporation.

When I was a small child, I had a vision of being a "scientist" when I grew up. At the age of fourteen, I played my first computer game and my vision for my future modified itself to include writing computer software. I am now a "computer scientist," if you believe the piece of paper I received when I finished college.

People create new visions daily. Visions for life, visions for love, visions for their families. Churches have visions, governments have visions, and entire countries have visions. Invariably, these visions are for some form of improvement: growing a company, having a fulfilling job, making a wonderful family, and so on. We plan these things, sometimes we write them down, and we expend considerable effort turning the visions into a reality. Why then, when it comes to our health, do we have no vision?

We watch television, eating our cookies, snack cakes, chips, burgers, candy, and ice cream, glassily staring at the moving images. We're more content to *watch* a sporting event than to participate in one. We load our systems with artificial colors and flavors, once-natural foods that have been so processed they need to be "enriched" to have even the slightest nutritional value, saturated fats, and that all-time favorite of mine, partially hydrogenated vegetable oil.

Is it any wonder we're fat? That obesity is reaching epidemic proportions? That heart disease, cancer, and diabetes are running rampant? Scientists have shown time and time again that though there are *some* genetic predispositions toward these diseases, one's lifestyle can greatly affect his or her chances of getting one of them.

We don't plan to do this. No one sits around and says, "My vision for my life is to weigh over 350 pounds by the time I'm 30, and if I'm lucky, to pop off from a heart attack by 40 or at the very latest, complications from diabetes by 45." I know I had no such plans. But, by not having a vision for my health, I was guaranteeing the ultimate failure with regards to it: death, or at the very least suffering and dismemberment.

Yuck.

March 31

Before I had a mental transformation last May, I was prone to buy things at the grocery store that weren't on the list I took with me each week. On a typical week, I'd pick up a box or two of Little Debbie cakes, maybe some Oreos or chocolate chip cookies, a couple of bags of chips, and two pints of Ben and Jerry's ice cream.

Things are different now.

I went to get groceries this morning, as I do every Saturday morning, and as usual I bought some things that weren't on the list. It was on the way home that I realized just *how* different I am now than I was almost a year ago. How different? The items I bought today that weren't on my list: three bananas, a cantaloupe, and a bag of organic puffed wheat.

April 2001

243 – 234 *pounds*

April 2

Live like a fit and healthy person, become a fit and healthy person. Live like a super-fat person, become a super-fat person. The choice is yours, right now.

Living like a fit person sounds like a simplistic rule, but really isn't. When it's time to eat, for example, I ask a question: "As a fit and healthy man, is this something I want to put in my body?" If the answer is yes, I eat it. If it's no, I don't. See what I mean? I lapse in my questioning from time to time, and eat things I wouldn't normally have, but the overall trend is good. Remember, we're aiming for progress, not perfection.

As a short side note, the question above is functionally equivalent to one I've used here before with regards to eating. The other question is "Will this food help me or hurt me?" Basically the same question, only phrased differently. It all boils down to the idea that if I were a fit and healthy man, there are certain foods I would eat, and certain foods I would not. I'm suggesting we just think before we eat.

I believe to my core that just by being mindful of what's going in, I don't have to focus so much on counting calories or anything along those lines. This has worked so far, but I won't know 100% until I get done with all this, to see how close I was.

When it comes to physical activity, I endeavor to live like that fit and healthy man I see in my head. I exercise like him, not like a fat man – and though I sometimes pay a price in soreness, I think it's worth it. The more I live like that man, the more I feel and look like him.

And soon, I'll find that I have become him.

April 6

I went mountain-bike riding yesterday, down by the river and it was just plain awesome. I even did a little off-roading on the bike, and managed to get quite muddy.

I felt like a real athlete, briefly.

I also climbed on the jungle gym at a playground by the bike path, and went down the tornado slide. That kicked ass.

I put a trailer hitch on my Jeep today and bought a hitch-mount bike rack, so I don't have to wrestle the bike into the cargo area. Slowly but surely I feel like I'm turning into an outdoor person, much like when I was a small, mostly-thin child.

And I like it.

As I've said on many occasions, when I look into the mirror, I don't see the Fred that's really there. I see the one who exists in my head, the new Fred, the one I decided I wanted to be roughly ten months ago. When I think about myself, I see this new man, and not the old.

This process is called "visualization," and it works hand in hand with the idea I talked about last time – living "as if" you're the person you want to be. As long as you're living like that person, why not go ahead and see yourself as that person while you're on your way?

Remember, I believe that transforming oneself is more a mental thing than a physical thing. Mold the mind, and the body will follow. Therefore, if you live like the person you want to be, and see yourself as that person, you will become that person.

Think about it for a minute.

When I was riding the greenway by the river yesterday, I came to a point where the greenway crossed a small bridge going over the creek. At each end of this bridge there was a metal post sunk into the concrete, right in the middle of the path. To the left side of the path was a 10-foot drop into shallow, rocky water. To the right side was one of the busier roads in Huntsville.

As I approached the bridge, I got obsessed with that metal post. I could see the collision in my head. *Don't hit the post,* I thought, *because if you fall left, you can go over the little fence and onto the rocks below, and if you go right, you could become road kill. Stay away from the damn post!*

I almost hit the post.

Fortunately, I realized at the last second that I was doing exactly what I preach about, headed directly for the dreaded post, and narrowly circumvented it (to the left, if you're curious). Focus on being fat, lazy, whatever, and fat, lazy, whatever you will be. Focus on being a fit and healthy person, and watch yourself become one.

April 9

I haven't been wearing my expensive $75 helmet when I ride my bike. Why not? Because it looked funny on my head, sort of like the whole little cowboy hat on the Mr. Potato Head thing, sitting way up high and making me look more dorky than normal. I assumed it was because I have a big head. I was wrong.

Moron that I am, I was wearing it backwards all along.

April 11

Somewhere, I read a statistic, which effectively stated that 90% of the people who attempt to lose weight fail. In my experience, I've noticed that something like 90% of all the people who "diet" are doing it in order to fit into a dress, see an old friend, go to a high school reunion, or something similar.

I see a correlation here. As long as you're attempting to drop excess weight for any reason other than for you alone, you're pretty much destined to become one of the aforementioned statistics. The truly lasting change must come from within, not from without.

❧

There is no reality in this life; there is only perception. Reality for you is just your perception of the events around you, because you have total control over your perceptions. You choose to perceive things however you desire. As a result, you create your own reality.

I choose to perceive what I'm doing as a simple thing, not difficult at all, and certainly not a struggle, a war, a battle, or any of the other metaphors used to describe the process of taking charge of one's life and getting rid of extra fat. As a result, my reality is this: dropping weight, getting rid of diabetes, becoming healthy – all of these are simple, because I choose for them to be. Not eating the Oreos and fried chicken I once ate is easy, because I choose to perceive it that way.

Regularly, people refer to my "struggle" to get rid of my excess weight, and then get incensed when I comment that it was not (is not) a struggle at all. I cannot help that (in a more smug mood, I might comment that they *choose* to *perceive* my answer as untruthful), because I choose to not view what I'm doing in that way. I view it as: (a) something to just *do*, and (b) something that's not hard at all.

And guess what? For me, it isn't.

You can choose to perceive it as difficult, and thus make it difficult for you, or you can choose to perceive it as something that is trivial, and make it so. Which do you choose?

April 14

Recently, I've been thinking a lot about the idea of "maintenance" with regards to weight. Plainly stated, I don't hold for it. Maintenance implies some sort of lifelong struggle to maintain a specific weight. I don't need to go into how I feel about looking at this process as a struggle – you can check out my last entry for my thoughts on that.

Way back in early June last year, while I was still performing all my mental programming, I made a decision to live like a different man. Specifically, I decided to live like a fit and healthy man, and slowly but surely, I'm becoming that man. When I reach my goal, I will *be* that man, and I will continue to live like the man I want to be.

If that's what I'm doing, why is there any need to "maintain" anything?

I'll simply continue to live like the new man, and I will remain that man. No struggles, no worries, no nothing. I do realize right now that I'm not perfect, and I will probably have to do a bit of tweaking when I get there (if not before) because the amount of food I eat and exercise I do is based on an idea I have in my head, and may be off slightly from reality (or my perception of it, anyway). I may need to eat more when I weigh 190, I may need to eat less. I'm reasonably sure I am doing what is right now, and that I won't have to make any significant tweaks.

Call that maintenance if you want – I would rather not.

April 16

I realized today that I've now dropped more weight than my 12-year-old daughter weighs. Damn, I was fat.

April 24

I took a random sample test of my almost-resting heart rate last night and found it to be 68 beats per minute. The average for a male is 72, and mine used to be in the 90's. If you don't know, lower is better – the lower it is, the more athletic (boy, that word sounds funny in a sentence about me) you are.

What this means, of course, is that after almost 11 months of pushing myself physically every single day, I'm in slightly better shape than the average person.

Jeez.

April 27

For almost 20 years, America has been obsessed with fat. We look for fat-free and low-fat foods, and stuff our faces with them because of this fat obsession. *Fat is evil,* we think to ourselves, because that's what we've been told.

Let me clear something up: fat is *not* evil. A calorie is a calorie, regardless of its source. Granted, fat has more calories per gram than anything else, but that just makes it energy-packed, not evil. My internal pressure on this subject has been building, but it culminated today when I got an email from an online friend sending me some "diet tips." The particular tip that bothered me was the suggestion to eat pita bread instead of a tortilla, because the pita has less fat grams. Same number of calories, but less fat.

What crap.

Here's the truth, plain and simple: to effectively drop weight, you have to burn more calories than you consume. Period. You can get your calories from fat, protein, carbohydrates, or even alcohol, should you want to. Since my focus is on health, I aim for getting a balance of foods (alcohol notwithstanding; I'm not a drinking man) because I think a balance of foods brings with it a balance of nutrition, and provides a terrific supply of nutrients and energy for my body.

Since America has become obsessed with the fat gram, our waists have ballooned until over 60% of the adult population is overweight. How could this be? We're eating less fat now (roughly 33% of our calories, down from 40% in the 70's) than we have recently. The answer probably is no surprise: we're eating more food, in part to compensate for eating less fat.

I can eat more of this, we think, *because it's reduced fat*.

Here's a question for you: when they took the fat out of the food, what did they replace it with? Sugar? Salt? Fillers?

Researchers at Stanford University did a study where they fed two groups of people diets identical in calories, fat, cholesterol, and protein. The difference between the diets is that one group got mostly "junk food" – SnackWell's cookies, fat-free and reduced fat snacks, and reduced fat lunch meats, for example – and the other group ate unprocessed foods. Both of the diets had about the same amount of sugar, but the first group's came from the snack foods and the second group's came from whole fruits.

The results? On the convenience food diet plasma triglycerides (fat in your blood) increased by 30%, while the whole-food group saw their plasma triglycerides decrease by 25%. What you eat matters.

❧

I found another interesting study today, done by the University of North Carolina. Did you know that in America, only 21.3% of adolescents take a gym class at least once a week? One out of five. And we wonder where all the fat grownups are coming from. It certainly isn't from that obesity gene we've all heard about, because as callous as it sounds, our gene pool didn't mutate that much in a generation.

Although it sounds like I'm opposed to reduced-fat and fat-free foods, I'm not. God knows I eat them too (particularly salad dressings). They're perfectly fine, in moderation, like everything else – and if you don't overdo them, they *can* help you drop weight. The secret is to not eat more just to compensate for less fat.

May 2001

233 – 231 *pounds*

May 2

I ate a candy bar today.

Not because I wanted it, or because I'm "slipping," but because I very nearly thought I was about to die, and it was the only thing quickly available to me.

It all started earlier today, while I was still at work. Things were slow and I wanted to move a bit, so I grabbed a co-worker and scampered out to the field behind our office to throw the Frisbee for a few minutes. Sometimes you just have to get away from the desk.

Today was a gorgeous day, a little over 80 degrees and wonderfully sunny. It was a little windy for the Frisbee, though, and that put a bit of a damper on the throwing. I spent a goodly part of the time chasing the Frisbee, but not actually running because the field is rocky and I didn't want to twist my ankle.

Things were great for about ten minutes then something really strange happened. The Frisbee was sailing toward me, nice and slow but a bit high. It floated lazily over my head, then made a semi-circle turn as it passed me and landed in the dry grass about 20 feet away. That's when my vision started darkening and closing in around the edges. I was suddenly dizzy as hell, and I think I very nearly passed out. I paused for a second with my eyes squeezed tightly shut, and the worst of the feeling passed. My vision cleared, and I walked over to the Frisbee. As I reached down for it I saw my hand quaking and shaking like a leaf in a high wind.

I ran through the things I figured could be wrong with me. *Dehydration?* No, I drink like a fish, and had consumed plenty of water over the course of the day. *Sunstroke*? Possibly, but I really wasn't out there long, and I wasn't overdoing it by any stretch of the imagination. The only thing I could settle on was low blood sugar, which I'm still torn about because I'd had a nice big lunch of spaghetti about 45 minutes before I went out to play.

So, I bought a candy bar with my shaky hands and ate it. I started feeling better within minutes, and feel fine now, except I'm still pretty tired. I checked my blood sugar when I got home, roughly 45 minutes after the Snickers, and it was 96. I'd assumed it would be higher, what with the sugar going into my system and everything, so as it stands, I'm going to assume I was just having a low blood sugar episode while I was playing Frisbee.

The diabetic has come a long way, baby.

May 6

Robyn, Danielle, and I are going back to Gatlinburg on May 24. We do love the place, and this trip has some extra significance. We're going for Memorial Day weekend, just like we did last year, and we're renting a house again, just like last year. The trip is, of course, significant, because it was the return from last year's trip that set off the chain of events that resulted in me being an entirely different man.

We're also going so we can celebrate my 34th birthday, which falls on that weekend. My birthday is on a Saturday this year, on the 26th, and I'm still bowled over by how different things are now. I have to say my prospects for a long life are definitely much greater this time around, and sometime before we leave, I want to write an entry comparing this birthday with my last one.

May 7

I went to JC Penney today, to buy some new 36-inch jeans. As I walked toward the door to go in, I looked up at the bank of reflective windows and caught sight of myself. I came to a complete stop there on the sidewalk, just looking.

Because I suddenly realized I wasn't fat at all.

Not by any *real* stretch of the imagination, anyway. Don't get me wrong, I wasn't thin by any means, but I wasn't fat, either. I was just a big guy, perfectly normal looking, and I was stunned. The man who's been living inside me is finally cracking out of the shell, and that is awesome. That man bought 2 pairs of 36-inch Levi's, 2 pairs of 36-inch Dockers shorts, and 2 XL cotton shirts. Only one X! Not two, not three, and certainly not the five X's I once wore.

Since the end of last May – less than a year ago – I've dropped my pants down by eighteen inches and dropped four X's off my shirt sizes.

May 11

I realized today that I'm becoming an active person, someone who enjoys moving outside the realm of simple exercise. I've started playing Frisbee quite a bit right before I leave work for the day, and just recently I've taken up doing various styles of pushups for fun, simply because I'm able. Matter of fact, not only can I now do pushups where my feet are higher than my head (like up on a desk, with my hands on the floor), I can even do clapping pushups (though my wife tells me my butt pokes comically high in the air when I do them), something I was never able to do, even when I was younger and not-really-fat. Several times a week I take afternoon bike rides for fun, often going seven to ten miles. I do all this in addition to my regular exercise I do when I first get out of bed each morning.

I'm actually looking forward to going on a mountain hike when we're in Gatlinburg in a couple of weeks, and my only real complaint about it is that we'll have to take the shorter and easier hike because out daughter will be with us. What I *really* want to do is take the 8-mile waterfall hike that's rated "strenuous" by the Park. I'd consider doing it alone, but I don't want to spend that much vacation time away from the family – we're only going to be there a couple of days. Funny, when you think about the trip to Gatlinburg last May, the one where I had to sit down and rest my ankles every couple of blocks on the strip.

It's nothing short of amazing that I can have days like yesterday, where I walk three and a half miles, play Frisbee for 20 minutes, work out with weights for 40 minutes, then go on a 10-mile bike ride, and not even feel tired when the day is over. I guess what it all boils down to is this: even if what I am now is a freak, I don't care.

I like it.

May 14

In my most recent blood sugar test at the doctor's office, my fasting blood sugar was 66. According to the nurse there, that's the absolute lowest number in the "normal" range. Who'd have thought I could go from being a big fat super-diabetic to being a not-so-fat, almost-hypoglycemic in less than a year?

May 15

I had another one of those pesky episodes today. You know, the one where I get all dizzy, weak, and shaky, and have to stop playing Frisbee. I ate a handful of Jelly Bellys and a fruit-n-grain bar and all was well, but I've been very sleepy ever since.

May 16

If we consider the whole/organic food section in the grocery store to be the "health food" section, what exactly does that make the rest of the food in the store?

May 17

I went to see my doctor today, to talk to her about my spells and whatnot. She thinks they're most likely my blood sugar, like I thought, but it's possible that it's actually my blood pressure, what with Frisbee involving all that bending down and such. We both agreed that it was odd that I can walk-jog, bicycle, or lift weights for 45 – 60 minutes at a time with no problems, but a little bit of Frisbee does that to me.

The solution is for me to keep an eye on it and see if I can discern a pattern. Even if it *is* low blood sugar, the only real solution is to wait for it to happen then eat some sugar.

Blood sugar is a big pain in the butt, for the record.

My heart rate, as measured by the nurse, was 60 beats per minute.

May 19

Thursday night, Robyn and I went to our daughter's school for a band concert, and the strangest thing happened. With all my positive thoughts and visualization, with seeing myself in the JC Penney window and realizing I'm not fat, and even with sitting there in my 36-inch pants and XL shirt, I felt like I was the fattest man in the place. In retrospect it's humorous, because I'm used to being the fattest guy in the place and now that I wasn't, I still felt like I was.

I know this, because I continually elbowed my wife, pointed someone out, and asked, "Am I fatter than him?" She would check the other guy out, then tell me I was nowhere close to being as big. Since I trust my wife, I believed her.

Mostly.

May 22

Often, we're at work doing our jobs when someone else in the office brings in a dessert-type dish and puts it out in the common area for all to enjoy. It sits out there calling to us, begging us to come to it, until we inevitably give in a go get a piece (or several, if no one's around). Why is that? What makes us suddenly turn from normal people into eating machines? Is the food evil? Are we weak?

We've all had these urges, and they're caused by any number of factors. One factor that has a real pull for me with regard to these urges is the idea of scarcity. We get worked up because we start thinking *there's only a little bit left, and if I don't have any right now, I don't know what I'll do*. We become agitated because we're starting to feel the mental pain we've created, and we end up filling our plates with about five times more than is healthy. So how do we change that?

First, recognize that the idea of scarcity is in your head. You've created that sense on your own; it's not external at all. This scarcity drives your desire through the roof. Once you recognize what you're doing, do something else. Interrupt the pattern of behavior you've fallen into, and your desire will drop almost immediately.

Once you're past the immediacy of having to have the food, you can use some more mind tricks to not only make the food less desirable, you can make it downright undesirable. For example, cookies sound pretty appealing, don't they? Cookies dipped in clam juice do *not* sound appealing. See what I mean? You can use other foods, or even the physical aspects of a food, to make something less appealing. Given a soft drink, you could imagine it warm and flat. See the grease from the top of a pizza lining your arteries. That cinnamon roll is probably not nearly as good with powdery green mold growing on it.

You can be as nice or as nasty as you like. I'm fond of incorporating vomit, feces, and insects into my visions, because they can change desire into disgust literally within a heartbeat. With a little practice, you can make this technique become second nature, and watch how much your urges decrease.

May 27

Dear Diary,

It's Sunday afternoon, and we just got back from our vacation to Gatlinburg, Tennessee, about two hours ago. What a great time we had, Diary! It's been so long since I had such fun I'd forgotten it was even possible to have so much. Our trip this year was so incredibly different from the one we took last year words cannot even begin to describe it.

But I shall try, Diary, I shall try.

We left home at about eleven o'clock in the morning. Our four-and-a-half hour trip took about six hours because of traffic problems in eastern Tennessee and because we stopped to eat lunch at Schlotzsky's on the way up. By the time we got to our rental house it was almost six o'clock so I grilled some small steaks and we had those, along with sweet potatoes and salad. Funny, Diary, we did the same thing last year, only I had two big steaks then, and my potato was loaded down with butter, sour cream, and cheese. We had cake for dessert last year, too.

We spent the rest of the night lounging around the house, and went to bed around ten because we were sleepy. I slept like a rock, without the problems breathing and snoring myself awake I had last year. Getting up bright and early, I drove down into town and took a brisk four-mile walk to get my blood going. Gatlinburg in the early morning is very pretty, but it was raining that Friday and I had to carry my umbrella with me.

After my walk I went back to the house and showered. I ate my oatmeal with mixed berries (and an apple for a little extra boost) and then we went back into town. We parked the car in the middle of town and set out. I remember last year well, because on the same Friday last year it was just Danielle and I. Robyn stayed at the house because she didn't feel like walking around in town. I don't blame her at all for that, because I had to stop every block and rest last year. My feet hurt too bad to walk more than that, and I would get out of breath. People just don't understand what it's like to lug around almost 400 pounds.

Things were different this time. All in all, my pedometer tells me I walked over twelve miles on Friday, and I wasn't a bit tired or sore the whole time! It's like I'm a new man, Diary, and I just love who I am now! I wondered if I'd be sore at all on Saturday when I got up, and I wasn't. I managed to cover over nine miles on my birthday.

That's a hell of a lot better than last year, Diary.

And the things I did. I played laser-tag for the first time ever. Twice. Running, jumping, and ducking, and I loved it. I went to a haunted theater, and I rode some amusement park rides, like the Tilt-A-Whirl. I even rode a merry-go-round (even though I looked like a fool), because I knew the horse would hold me now and not break off under my weight.

This year I rode the go-carts instead of just watching longingly from a distance. It's funny how I cannot shake the idea of being really fat. I made the attendant let me get into the go-cart before I paid, just to make sure I fit. I fit just fine and ended up telling him about the 140-pound monkey I've spent the last year slaying, mostly because of the look he gave me when I told him I wanted to make sure I wasn't too big for the go-cart.

We visited Ripley's Aquarium, which just opened, and it was great. I saw all kinds of neat things, but I really liked seeing all the sharks. I got to play with a horseshoe crab there, too. I played putt-putt golf, I rode a virtual roller coaster that spun me upside down, two other roller-coaster rides that didn't, and went to countless movies in theaters where the seats move. I even had an old-time picture made, Diary, my first ever. I was worried about the clothes being too small, but the pants were so big they almost fell off!

All in all, this was the best vacation of my entire adult life. I spent the whole time acting like a kid just because I can, and I cannot wait for our next vacation. Life is full of wonderful experiences now, Diary, and I'm happy to be here to experience them.

May 28

Here it is, May 28, 2001. It has been one year to the day since I found my pain, in the form of a rotting foot on television. With a year comes some reflection, and a look back at some of the ways life is different now.

- Today, I weigh 140 pounds less than last May 28. That's more than my child weighs, more than my mother weighs, and more than my sister weighs. It's almost 40% of my initial body weight of 371 pounds.
- My pants have moved from having a 54-inch waist to having a 36-inch one. My father, who weighs 174 pounds, wears 36-inch pants.
- My shirts, XXXXXL this time last year, are now XL.
- I'm no longer a diabetic. My fasting blood sugar has gone from the 180's to the 60's. Medicine is a thing of the past.
- I can buy all my clothes in any men's store, without having to look for a special fat man's store.
- I can trot up several flights of stairs, nonstop, without breathing hard at all. My heart doesn't even speed up.
- My resting heart rate, in the 90s one year ago, is now at 60.
- I have exercised 346 contiguous days now, and exercise an hour or more each day. This time last year I had to sit and rest my feet after walking a block.
- I have lots of visible muscles now.
- I can see my genitals again.
- My erections are bigger and firmer, and not prone to wither away like last year's.
- Sex lasts longer, and is much better. See above.
- I fit on amusement park rides now. Easily.
- I can ride a horse, because I no longer weigh too much.
- I don't avoid the camera any more.
- I can ride a bike again.

- I can run.
- I can play like a child.
- My gut, which once lightly touched the steering wheel of my Jeep when I drove, is more than six inches away from it now.
- My face looks normal again.
- I no longer snore, unless I fall asleep on my back.
- I sleep the night through, without having any disturbing apnea episodes where I stop breathing.
- I stay in bed about six hours a night, instead of the eight I used to.
- I don't have problems with yeast infections or boils any more.
- I can cut my own toenails.
- I fit in booths, theater seats, and the regular smock at the barber's.
- I wear t-shirts without being (too) concerned about my man-boobs.
- I love myself more each day.
- I can do multiple pushups, even with my feet above my head.
- I weigh what I did when I was 20 years old, and I'm in better shape than I've ever been in my life.
- My wife and daughter can both reach all the way around me at my largest point, with several inches to spare.
- I'm virtually pain-free now (unless I overdo it on the exercise, but that's a good pain).
- My total cholesterol is 119.
- My triglycerides are 76.
- I no longer get heartburn.
- I have a lap.
- I'm not embarrassed to be seen in public, and I don't mind running into people from my thinner past.

Most of all, I feel like I'm alive now, more alive than I've ever been, and I wouldn't trade that for anything.

May 31

I went to the grocery store last night to pick up some more salad and tuna (and some jelly beans, truth be told), and took the opportunity to jump on the blood pressure machine, to find my pulse. Fifty-four beats per minute.

June 2001

230 – 224 pounds

June 3

I went into my gym (what we call our extra room that's filled with exercise stuff; we're a pretentious lot) last night, because I was feeling a little hyper. I wanted to do some moving, and I could hear Billy Blanks calling my name through the door, wanting me to come do a little double time Tae Bo with him.

I turned on the big-screen TV we use for exercise videos (hey, I said we were pretentious) and reached for the Tae Bo Basic tape.

"Fred," Billy said from behind me, startling me and causing me to almost drop the tape.

I recovered, and turned to face him. "Billy? What're you doing here?" I asked.

"I'm here to remind you that you've been using that wimpy basic tape for almost ten months now. You know you were doing that tape back when you weighed more than 300 pounds. What's the problem?"

"I tried the advanced tape, Billy, and it kicked my butt. I'm scared to try it again!"

"You tried that tape months ago, Fred. Of course it kicked your butt! Now put that basic tape down, put in the advanced tape, and gimme some!"

So I did. I did 40 minutes of that tape, and I loved every single second.

June 4

People want a magic pill, something to just melt the built-up accumulation of years of unhealthy eating and exercise habits, and there's not one. They'll try grapefruit juice diets, diets consisting primarily of cabbage soup, various and sundry potions and pills containing stimulants, "fat blockers," and numerous other "solutions." Even when they recognize the folly of these things, they still try them out to "kick-start" their permanent change.

I'd like to take the high road here and laugh about these people, but the truth is, I too once felt like I needed something to help me with a little kick-start. I knew beyond the shadow of a doubt that if I could just find the one little thing to start the ball rolling, I'd be set and the weight would just fall off.

I never found it.

What I did find, however, is what I consider to be the universal truth of dropping weight: there's only one magic pill, and it's inside each one of us, not in a diet or a bottle. It starts with a decision to raise one's standards and to no longer live in the way they've been living.

It really is that simple, and it really is magical.

While I don't consider myself to be a success yet, I do consider myself to be well on the way, and I'm seeing the magic firsthand. I don't follow a particular program, except to exercise regularly and to eat mostly unprocessed foods, and that seems to be working pretty well for me. You, however, may be different. You might want the structure of something like Weight Watchers, or TOPS, or a diabetic exchange program. We're all different, and we can all arrive at the same destination by different – yet sensible – paths.

I'm leery of calling what I'm doing a "lifestyle change" (because that's the new buzzword dieters use), but I suppose that's what it is. I prefer to think of it as a mind-style change, sort of a new way of looking at things. I figure if I don't think of the way I'm living as "a program" or being "on the wagon," then there's no way I can ever go "off program" or "fall off the wagon." I eat to live, where I once lived to eat. Eating to live is just like it sounds: choosing a wide variety of nutrient-dense foods to provide adequate fuel for your body.

It is this same mind-style that lets me see what I'm doing as easy, not difficult, and definitely not as a war. It's why I don't rely on motivation, and why I don't hold for the idea of maintenance. Life is all about perceptions, and your reality is exactly what you perceive it to be. I choose to perceive mine as a simple process where I just live like the man I want to be, and I get to sit back and watch myself turn into that man.

June 8

This morning at work, while I was getting a glass of water from the cooler in the kitchen, my eye fell on a box of Cocoa Puffs, because that's a cereal I once loved. Emblazoned on the side of the box was the following statement:

Frosted Corn Puffs made with REAL COCOA*!*

Something about that statement disturbs me. Have we come so far in what we do to our food that we have to brag when we use a "real" ingredient?

❧

Regularly when I chat with people or talk via email, and even in the books I read, I see foods like desserts referred to as treats, as in "I'll let myself have a small piece of cheesecake from time to time as a treat."

I don't want to sound down on people, because sometimes I feel like I do that, but I want to make a simple statement or two that you can take or leave. The definition of the word "treat" (the noun, not the verb), according to the dictionary, is "an especially unexpected source of joy, delight, or amusement." Considering food – even certain foods – to be a "treat" creates an emotional attachment to that food, and if you're fat, perhaps an emotional attachment with food is not the best thing. Food is fuel – gasoline for the body – and not something we use to gratify ourselves.

Lest I sound holier than thou, I'm not suggesting food is not to be enjoyed, because I enjoy food a lot. All I'm suggesting is that most of the time (remember, aim for progress, not perfection), consider the fuel factor of a food before you consider the enjoyment factor of it.

June 16

It is completed. 365 consecutive days of exercise are behind me.

June 17

A metaphor is a figure of speech in which a word or phrase that literally denotes one kind of object used in place of another to suggest an analogy between them. We use metaphors all the time, and they help to shape our thoughts considerably. Consider the following statement: *I'm a lazy pig*. That's a metaphor. What about this one? *Oh my God, I'm such a big fat cow!* How do you think statements like these can affect your views about yourself?

June 19

I paid a visit to a plastic surgeon today to talk about my loose skin. He poked and prodded, rubbed his chin, played with my man-boobs quite a bit, then showed me two different procedures for my stomach and two different procedures for my man-boobs. The long and short of it is this: he can knock me out, insert a large and long tube up my penis the wrong way, slice and dice me, knock me out of working out for 4 to 6 weeks, leave me with big nasty scars, and still not be able to really fix everything.

He kept using a word that just sticks in my craw. Liposuction. As in "suck that fat right out, because your big fat lazy butt couldn't do it on your own." I don't want any liposuction, I don't want a catheter in my penis, I don't want to be put into a chemically-controlled coma, and I don't want to be bedridden for days on end, for something that's the doctor seemed to say wasn't even going to fix it all. To hell with that, I say.

Interestingly, the doctor was fascinated by the fact that Robyn and I have done what we have without any invasive surgical procedures, and he seemed to really enjoy hearing the rotting foot story. He told me he just bought *Sugar Busters* a couple of weeks ago.

"Maybe that'll help me," he said on his way out the door.

I wondered why he couldn't just liposuck himself, since he seemed to want to liposuck me so bad.

June 21

I don't like someone telling me something cannot be done. That mentality bugs me, and I seem to be hearing it a lot these days:

It's impossible to quit smoking and not gain weight, people say.

Have I mentioned recently that I put my cigarettes down for good at the beginning of January, roughly 45 pounds ago, without picking them up again or gaining a pound?

You cannot lose weight without ____________ *(add your own fad diet, chemical, or surgical procedure name)*, they reiterate.

I beg to differ.

You cannot maintain your new weight without keeping a close eye on everything you eat, they whisper.

Watch me.

Following that thought, perhaps the reason that over 90% of people who attempt to drop weight fail, either in dropping it or in keeping it off, because they all have the same set of limiting beliefs. These beliefs include, but are not limited to:

Losing weight is so hard. *It's a war, a battle, a struggle, a fight, and it's bloody.*

No, it's not. It's what you choose to believe it is. Period. I choose to see it as a great adventure, and guess what? For me, that's what it is. Not because I'm special or because there's something magical, but because I choose to look at it that way.

Maintaining a drop in weight is the hardest part.

More crap. If I continue to live the way I'm living, I'm going to continue being the man I want to be. If you think I'm going to suddenly start wolfing down bags of Oreos and spending all my time sitting on my newly-thinned ass when I'm no longer fat, then you haven't been reading very carefully.

I'm too (old, fat, lazy, fill in the blank) to change.

Never! What you are is completely in your hands. You can be anyone you want to, and if you put your mind to it, nothing can stop you from being your all.

It's not that easy, Fred.

Yes, it is. Stop limiting yourself. You can be free from the limiting beliefs you're holding if you just let them go. That's all it takes.

June 22

In the world of computers, one company is the king. Many people love this company, and many people hate it. It is Microsoft, and it recently had a series of advertisements featuring a question that begs exploration.

Where do you want to go today?

That's a good question with regards to computers, but if we take it out of the context of computers and move it into the context of our lives, and specifically our weight/health, it suddenly takes on a whole new meaning.

Where do YOU want to go today?

Do you want to go nowhere, health-wise? Do you want today to be like the other days in your past, where you just "get by," and don't improve yourself in some small way? Or do you want to take charge of your life, living it to the fullest and pushing yourself to new heights of strength, endurance, and vitality? The choice is entirely yours.

Where do you want to GO today?

If you're not advancing, you're retreating. You can move forward, and make your health better and better, or you can move backwards, watching it decline. You hold your own destiny in your hands; you're the driver. Believe you me, if you don't want to do the driving in your life, someone else does, and it may not be the person you want.

Where do you want to go TODAY?

Are you worth the effort? I think you are, but what I think isn't really important. What do you think? Do you want to live life or let life live you? You can do it now, today, or you can put it off until tomorrow. Again.

Let's modify it a little, shall we?

Who do you want to be today?

Interesting question, isn't it? Who *do* you want to be? Do you want to be the same old person you've always been, sitting around your house and letting food control you? Or would you rather be the one in charge, seizing each day by the horns and living life to your fullest potential?

It's just a matter of choice, really. You can choose to take control of your life and transform yourself from what you are into what you know you can be, or you can stay hidden inside a cocoon of fat ar of what real life is like. The choice is yours.

Who do you want to be today?

June 24

According to the dictionary, the third definition of the word "standard" is "something established by authority, custom, or general consent as a model or example." Synonyms for this word include criterion, gauge, and yardstick. We measure ourselves by our standards, and they run our lives. At any given point in time we're living by our standards. What are your standards with regards to your health?

There was a time in the not too distant past when my standards for myself were nonexistent. I was content to sit back and watch life pass me by while I kept one hand on the remote and the other in a bag of cookies. My standards (or lack thereof) got my weight up to almost 400 pounds, made me a diabetic, and would've ultimately killed me, most likely at a young age. I couldn't walk up the stairs in my house without breathing hard, amusement park rides were a thing of the past, and if I wanted to fly anywhere I had to either buy two seats or go first class.

What are your standards? Do they exist? Are your standards for yourself low or high?

One of the easiest ways in the world to transform your health and fitness is to raise your standards. I've talked a lot over the last year about the power of decisions, and the ultimate decision comes when you decide to raise your standards for yourself. For me, I decided I was no longer willing to let life pass me by while I ate my way into an early grave. I raised my standards dramatically when I made that decision, and they've continued to rise over the last 13 months. Some of those health standards are:

- I will take responsibility for my life and what I do. Whatever I put into my body is my choice.
- I choose to eat mostly whole and healthful foods, and I refuse to feel bad or guilty if I do choose something unhealthy.
- I will do whatever it takes to make myself into the fit and healthy man I want to be.
- I will no longer poison myself with tobacco use.

- I will make sure to move my butt regularly, and to strive for continual improvement in my exercise.
- I will regularly evaluate my standards, and raise them whenever I've become complacent.

Think about your own standards for a bit then find one in particular you can raise. What are the benefits you'd get from raising that one little standard?

June 25

Each day you're on this earth you have a new opportunity to improve your health. One more chance to change things before it's too late. What do you choose to do with this day?

Do you choose to put wholesome and healthful foods into your body, or do you choose junk because it's just "so much easier?" There's a reason they're called convenience foods, you know. Are you worth the extra time it takes to prepare food that your body can effectively utilize? Do you choose to move and improve your body by being active, or are you "too tired" and "don't have enough time?" Nothing creates boundless energy like being in good health and in good shape, and we all have enough time if we really want it. How much time do you spend watching TV?

They're called excuses and they'll kill you if you let them. We use them to remove blame from ourselves and to become victims. Victims of food, emotions, society, other people, you name it. They allow us to say, in essence, "I cannot help it if I'm fat; it isn't my fault." I'm here to shed some light for you. Chances are good it *is* your fault. In the vast majority of cases, one gets fat because they are living like a fat person, not because of some external source. We choose to live like fat people, and fat people we become.

But I'm not here to put people down; I'm here to tell you there's hope.

You don't have to be a victim any more. All you have to do is realize that you are the one in charge. Not food, not emotions, not any other person. You. Realizing that you're in control gives you unlimited power to take charge of your life, and decide to stop living the life that got you where you are.

You can change, you know, whether you think it's possible or not. You don't need to be "motivated" to do it, you don't need a "support group" to do it, and you don't need a special diet, pill, or operation. All you need is you. What do you choose to do with this day?

June 27

Everywhere you look, you're inundated with advertising for products designed to help you drop weight. From Jared and his Subway sandwiches to Fergie and her point-counting friends at Weight Watchers, you cannot miss them. You turn on the radio and hear the DJ hawking Metabolife, or hear ads for Dexatrim Natural.

Richard Simmons, Jenny Craig, FormYou3, Physician's Weight Loss Centers, Herbalife, NutriSystem, Beverly Hills International, The Hollywood Diet, TrimSpa, FatWhacker, Chito-san, Xenical, Meridia, Aloha Weight Loss, Atkins, The Zone, Pritikin, Ornish, The Grapefruit Diet, The Cabbage Soup Diet, The Rotation Diet, The T-factor Diet, L.A. Weightloss, Dr. Bernstein.

And in every one of these advertisements, down in the corner, in very small letters, are three words: *Results not typical*. Harmless little words, aren't they? They sit down there in the corner, quietly hoping you'll miss them, that you'll just cough up some of your money for the product being touted.

I'm here to shed some light on these words.

Of *course* the results in the pictures aren't typical. If the ads wanted to show some typical results, they'd have pictures where the "after" shot had someone a little (or perhaps a lot) fatter than the one in the "before" picture. Advertisers don't want you to see that. If you did, you probably wouldn't pony up the cash.

A question begs answering: why are the typical results of the programs listed above so horrendous? The typical results are so bad because we want to turn our fat problem over to something or someone else.

I can have this pizza, we think, *I took a Xenical earlier this morning, and it'll move the evil fat right on through me*.

Xenical won't fix the problem, friend. Nor will any of the others listed above. Sure, they'll all work a little – and maybe even a lot. Until you stop using them, that is. Then watch your pounds come back, probably with a few friends.

You cannot rely on anything other than you. You have the magic; you have the power – not any diet, pill, or surgery. You also have a choice in the matter. Do you want to try yet another "program," in hopes that it will be the one, or do you want to grab life by the proverbial balls and take charge of it?

You have the choice to eat that cupcake and those Doritos. You also have the choice to stop eating them. It really is that simple, no matter what any dieters, doctors, or advertisers tell you. I've been there – am still there, for that matter – and I know just how simple it is.

How badly do you want it?

June 29

A large part of a successful transformation from fat to fit is mental. Obviously there are physical portions – God knows you cannot just will a physical change to occur, you actually have to take a little action – but it's a mostly mental process. Think and act like a fat person, and stay a fat person. Think and act like a healthy and fit person, and become one. I try to keep the main focus of this book on that mental process.

As such, I don't focus a whole lot on nutrition, because I believe that we have an instinctive idea of what's good for us and what's not. I'm not terribly concerned with what I eat, as long as I know most of it is unprocessed (in general, plenty of fruits, grains, and veggies, along with quality proteins and fats). I specifically try to stay away from discussing specifics of the dietary side because no one can seem to make up their minds about what's right to eat.

Dr. Atkins tells us protein is most important, the Zone tells us we need a 30-30-40 balance of our foods, and the official U.S. government pyramid places its emphasis on carbohydrates. My bodybuilding books tell me to eat more protein to build muscle; my personal trainer books tell me the body uses carbohydrates to do that.

Be sensible: Eat natural foods in reasonable quantities, and work your body regularly. Don't over-think things.

June 30

The alarm rings, and you wake up slapping it off.

Get up and work out, or go back to sleep? your mind asks.

It's time for a decision. You may decide to get up and work out, you may decide to go back to sleep. That's not important for the purposes of this example.

What is important is this: whether you exercise or go back to sleep, you probably don't give your decision a second thought, but rather make it mindlessly and go on your way. All too often, we make the decisions in our lives without taking the time to mull them over. We are unaware of what we're doing most of the time, and it is that sort of thinking that leads to weighing almost 400 pounds, being a diabetic, and sitting on the couch munching on some Little Debbie snack cakes.

Decisions are important. Take time to think about things before you act. Don't take an eternity, just take a few seconds and mull over the options. Sometimes you'll find that you make the same decision you would've made mindlessly, sometimes you'll make a different decision. However, you'll be aware of what you are doing and your reasons behind it, which is good, because not only will you learn more about yourself, you'll learn more about your own motivations.

July 2001

224 – 220 pounds

July 2

Imagine making any of the following statements during the course of a conversation:

- "I don't have time to bathe every day."
- "The bathroom's too far out of the way to brush my teeth regularly."
- "I can't afford to wash my hair."
- "Taking a shower makes me too tired."
- "Brushing my teeth makes me too sore."
- "I'm too old to bathe."
- "I'm too fat to floss."
- "Washing my hair is too boring."
- "None of my friends shower regularly."
- "I can't wash my hair, I'm having my period."

Ludicrous, aren't they? I cannot imagine many, if any, people making comments like the ones above. But, make a few minor changes to each statement and they suddenly sound familiar, perhaps too familiar:

- "I don't have time to exercise every day."
- "The gym's too far out of the way to go there regularly."
- "I can't afford exercise equipment."
- "Working out makes me too tired."
- "Exercise makes me too sore."
- "I'm too old to lift weights."
- "I'm too fat to exercise."
- "Exercise is too boring."

- "None of my friends work out regularly."
- "I can't exercise, I'm having my period."

Physical activity is one of the most important things we can do for ourselves, yet the vast majority of us do it rarely, if at all. Why is that? Why don't we care more for our physical selves?

Mostly, it's simply because we don't think about it. And if we *do* think about it, many of us – particularly those who've been fat and out of shape for a long time – have pain linked to the idea. Since we avoid that which we perceive as pain, we avoid physical exertion and make our paltry excuses. No one can make excuses like a fat person.

Since we're so good at it, I'd like to make a novel suggestion. What if we make excuses to exercise instead of excuses to not exercise? Here are a few I came up with:

- "Working out makes me feel good about myself."
- "Lifting weights makes me feel stronger and more powerful."
- "Exercise outdoors gives me good time alone, thinking."
- "My spirit is refreshed when I work out."
- "Exercise lets me challenge myself regularly."

Did you exercise today?

July 4

People regularly make comments to me like, "You can't tell me you never hear a candy bar calling your name" or, "We're not all perfect like you are, Fred." I need to clarify something.

I'm not perfect, and I'm not making any attempt to be. Candy bars do call to me from time to time, and you know what? I either eat them or I don't, and I don't look back. As I've said before, I basically ask myself a simple question when I am presented with food: if I were a fit and healthy 190-pound man, would I eat this? If the answer is "yes," I eat it, and if it's "no," I don't. Fit and healthy men *do* eat candy bars on occasion, just not every day. Those fat and unhealthy 371-pound men, however, are the ones who do that.

I don't sit around and berate myself if I make less than optimal choices, and I don't write about it here, because the purpose of this journal is to *not* to obsess over the specifics, but to focus on a not-so-standard way of looking at the process of transforming from fat to fit.

❧

Today is the 4th of July, and in the United States we celebrate because it marks the anniversary of our declaration of independence from England 225 years ago.

You can be free, you know. All you have to do is declare your own independence from your limiting beliefs. Imagine the freedom of discarding some – or all – of the following beliefs:

- Losing weight is difficult, some big "war" where you fight against yourself or food.
- Past failures at losing weight dictate your future performance.
- You can only "try" to change yourself, with no guarantees.
- You're addicted to (insert your favorite food here).
- You cannot lose weight, so you'll just stay fat.
- You don't have any "willpower."
- Exercise is a chore.

Freedom. It's a mighty fine thing, and it's yours for the taking. You don't even have to start another war to get it, you just have to decide once and for all you want it more than anything else.

July 5

If you look on the website of the U.S. Securities and Exchange Commission, you'll find an interesting statement regarding mutual fund investing:

"This year's top-performing funds aren't necessarily going to be next year's best performers. That's why the SEC requires funds to tell investors that a fund's past performance does not necessarily predict future results."

Let's look briefly at a corollary statement, prepared by yours truly:

"Last year's health failures aren't necessarily going to be this year's poor performers. That's why the FEC (fat eradication committee) requires the fat man to tell readers that their past performance does not necessarily predict future results."

It's a very liberating thought, isn't it? No matter how many times you've tried and failed to change yourself in the past, that has exactly no bearing on anything you do in the future.

In financial investing, one generally looks at long-term results rather than the short term. There's a beautiful process in investing called "compounding interest," and it can work true monetary miracles. Compounding interest means that as you invest, you earn money on your investment. The money you earn in turn earns money, and starts a snowball effect so that after a certain length of time and with a certain investment, you meet your financial goals.

Your life is no different. It's an investment, and good health has its own compounding interest. Make a small investment with your time in regular exercise, and you can increase your life span by decades because of the cumulative effects. Start eating just a little bit less at each meal, and watch your weight loss snowball into 10, 20, 100, 200 pounds gone over time. It's a true miracle, and it's entirely within your grasp.

Invest in yourself. You're worth it.

July 9

My weight is up two pounds from last week, my first gain since I started all this way back in May of last year. Had this happened a year ago I'd be losing my mind right now, but frankly I'm not concerned.

Regularly I'm asked questions like "I weighed 140 this morning, and now I weigh 145. How can I gain 5 pounds in a *day*?" or "Yesterday I weighed 163 and today I weighed 170. How can that happen?" As always, I'm here with answers.

For the first question, the food you eat and the liquids you drink have weight. Sometimes we forget that. But, drinking a 32-oz glass of water is like strapping on a 2-pound weight, at least for a while. The same thing goes for what you're eating: it immediately adds weight to you, and that weight gradually goes away as you digest, burn the food for fuel, and eliminate.

The second question is one that can be more troublesome. Partly it can be explained with the items from the previous paragraph, but there's a second issue we tend to forget about. It's this that I'm pretty sure has happened to me. Spicy and salty foods can cause your body to hold water for several days after you eat them.

Friday morning, I weighed 222 pounds, down a pound from Monday's weight of 223. Friday night, Robyn and I went to a Mexican restaurant we'd never been to, and I ate lots of salty and spicy foods. Saturday morning, I weighed 224 pounds. This was to be expected, because Friday night's food was still working through my system. I did my normal thing all day Saturday, and when I weighed Sunday morning guess what?

Two hundred and thirty one pounds, the scales told me.

That's an increase of seven pounds in a single day, a physical impossibility, particularly since I didn't eat an extra 24,500 calories on Saturday. See what happened? The Mexican food from Friday night caused my body to grab water all day Saturday, and the results of that showed up on Sunday. They're still showing up today, since I weigh 225.

And here's the best part: even if I did gain two pounds this week, so what? Don't obsess over the details; watch the overall trend. If things are generally moving the direction you want them to, one blip won't kill you. It's a reversal of the trend you want to watch out for.

This is one of the reasons I weigh daily rather than weekly or monthly. I can watch my weight's trend, and I don't get any nasty surprises that way. Fluctuations are perfectly normal, and to be expected.

July 13

I didn't want to see a movie anyway, at the thought of squeezing into one of those tiny theater seats.

I like sitting in first class, when paying the extra money to upgrade, so you can fit in the seat.

Amusement parks are for kids, at the prospect of getting on a roller coaster and having the bar catch on your gut.

My *ankle's been hurting, I'd better take the elevator*, when a staircase presents itself.

Denial. It's such a small word, but has such a big meaning. Denial is a refusal to admit the truth or reality about a situation. We spend our lives in denial of our fatness, and we pay the ultimate price with diabetes, heart disease, arthritis, and a plethora of other side effects. Ultimately those side effects will most likely lead to an untimely and painful death.

Who wants that?

I'm calling it denial, but it's really lying. I spent 33 years lying to myself, making statements just like the ones above so I didn't have to face the pain of being a fat and lazy man who cared so little for himself that he allowed his weight to edge up to almost 400 pounds. My guess is that if you're reading this, you've spent some time lying to yourself, too – maybe not as much as I did, maybe even more.

You can end the denial right now. Admit that you've not made the wisest choices in your past. It's quite liberating, actually, and can be life changing. The choice is in your hands: resolve to be truthful yourself from this point forward, then let it go. There's no reason to agonize over what you've done in the past. It's over and done, release it. If you stay focused on what you've done in the past, you cannot fully focus on what you're doing for your future. Remember what I said just a few days ago about investments and investing in yourself? We're not looking for the instant payoff (stuffing our faces), because when we choose that the long-term outlook sucks. We're aiming for the future payoff, and taking actions today that affect our lives tomorrow.

Be true to yourself, and let the truth set you free.

July 18

Want to drop extra pounds without giving up your favorite foods?

Want to be able to eat cake and candy if you choose?

Are you sick of fad diets that promise miracles and cost lots of money?

Have you dieted, exercised, sweated to the oldies, counted your points, had high fat / low fat / no fat food – all with no results?

I have a great secret I've discovered after years and years of expensive research, and I'm willing to share it with you. You can use this secret to ultimately eat more than you ever dreamed, and still not gain a pound!

But wait, there's more!

Not only do you get ALL THIS, if you order now, I'll even throw in a FREE copy of the URL to my website – A FIVE HUNDRED DOLLAR VALUE – absolutely FREE!

Right now, you're probably saying to yourself, "How much does he want? What can I pay to get this secret? Whatever he's asking, it cannot be enough!"

You've probably seen similar secrets selling for $100, $200, even $500, but I'm here to give you this amazing secret without charging you a single dime!

Are you ready for the secret yet? Operators are standing by to take your order!

The secret is: muscle.

One pound of muscle burns up to 50 calories a day in the human body. Know what fat does? It just sits there. Muscle is an active tissue; fat is a passive tissue.

If you want to eat more food, the solution's simple: add a few pounds of muscle mass. No, I'm not kidding. You don't have to get all bulky, unless you want to get all bulky. Build muscle, and eat more. It really is that simple.

July 19

I eat more now than I did this time last year.

Did you hear that? I'm eating more in the low 220's than I did this time last year when I weighed in the low 320's, in no small part due to the muscle mass I've added. And here's the killer: I eat more now, and my weight is *still* going down.

Muscle. It does a body good.

July 24

America has become the land of instant gratification in recent years. We've become hooked on getting anything we want right now, from food at McDonald's on every corner to overnight delivery of anything to anywhere via Federal Express. We want things, we want them immediately, and we'll do anything to get them – at any price.

Enter the diet industry. Americans spend thirty billion dollars a year in the pursuit of instant weight-loss gratification. Don't believe me? Scan the classifieds section of your newspaper, check your email, or look on an auction web site. You'll find a plethora of claims like "lose 90 pounds in 2 months!" Don't fall for the hype. No matter what advertisers tell you, there's no magic pill, there's no quick fix to getting rid of extra fat – unless you want to try something silly, stupid, or dangerous. It took you *years* to get where you are, and you expect to get thin and healthy in a week?

Don't be a sheep for the weight-loss industry. If you want the "secret" to dropping weight, getting fit, and being downright full of life (though, truth be told, people often tell me there's something else I'm full of), I'll tell you, and I'll do it for free. Lean in close, and I'll whisper it in your ear. Are you ready?

Eat less. Move more.

I'm serious. I know it sounds smug and facetious and I'm saying it tongue-in-cheek, but it's ultimately true. For the vast majority of people, it's a simple equation: use more energy than you consume, and you will drop excess weight. Period.

In physics, power is defined as work over time. In a personal sense power is fitness, vitality, pure energy and health, and the only way to get it is to expend effort consistently over time. That's what I want out of life – true power.

The quick fix is rarely permanent, and often leads to poor health and fitness. If that's what you want, go buy some of those pills.

July 25

I had to go down to the insurance office today to sign paperwork on homeowner's insurance for our new house. Not so fun in and of itself, but I haven't been in the insurance agent's office for two years. My original agent died, and I was meeting my new agent for the very first time today. Clara, the intrepid assistant, has been working there forever, though, and she and I always got along well when my old agent was alive.

See where this one's going already?

I walked in, and my new agent and Clara were sitting at Clara's desk, waiting for me because I'd just called and told them I'd be right there. I smiled brightly at Clara as I came through the door.

Clara looked up at me and smiled, with nary a flicker of recognition in her eyes.

"May I help you?" she asked.

"Um, I'm here to see Kari," I said, my smile faltering slightly as I puzzled over how Clara could've forgotten me.

"Fred Anderson?" Kari asked, standing and holding out her hand.

Clara's brow wrinkled in concentration, but she didn't say anything. Kari shook my hand then led me back to her office. We left Clara blinking after us, looking dazed and somewhat confused.

My name was misspelled on the insurance policy, so Kari had to call Clara back, in order to get a new copy prepared. To make a long story short, Clara had made the connection and wanted to know all about what I'd done. Having people you know not recognize you is a strange feeling.

July 26

Yesterday, I was on the phone with one of my customers, and he asked about my progress. One thing led to another, and we started talking about fitness. Over the course of our conversation, we discussed how our fitness ideals had changed as our fitness levels had changed (this customer started exercising regularly and rigorously early this year, and is getting into extremely good shape).

Ultimately I said the following: "I think I'll be at the right level of fitness when I can do whatever I want without passing out or having a heart attack."

Fast forward to this morning. Recently, I've kicked up the speed of my walking about a half-mile per hour or so, to get a more intense workout. This morning, about a tenth of a mile away from my house, I got some serious pain in my right upper inner thigh, which made me start gimping and hobbling pretty badly. I believe the new hyper-walking might've caused it, but then again, I could have just been a little stiff.

I didn't want to turn around and go home so I kept walking, slightly slower, in hopes that I'd walk it off. Sure enough I did, after about a hundred or so steps. I continued walking happily. Until, that is, the pain came back with a vengeance when I was about three-tenths of a mile from home.

Hmmm, I thought, *I can try a little running. That utilizes muscles differently and might not hurt.* So I ran a little and sure enough, running didn't hurt. I went back to walking after a very short distance, and by the time I'd gotten about a half-mile from home, the pain was back. This time, however, it was practically excruciating – enough to actually cause me a little concern. So I started running again.

All in all, I ran about two miles, nonstop, and I only ended up stopping because my left leg started hurting a little, ironically in the same place my right one did. That, my friends, is what I'm talking about with regards to fitness. I ran, because I wanted to, and I ran a good long time without ever really getting tired.

And that rocks.

❧

Yesterday, my grandmother died. It was expected, because she'd been fading for the last several months. That's neither here nor there, though, what's important is this: my grandmother was 93 years old (within a few months of 94, truth be told), living alone, and pretty much taking care of herself right up until about 4 months ago.

She was ninety-three years old and in great health almost to the very end.

She spent her life eating fresh vegetables from her garden, fresh fruits from the farmer's market, fresh meat she raised and killed, and plenty of "taboo" foods like eggs and butter. She cooked with lard.

She was ninety-three years old, and in great health almost to the very end.

Know what else she did, right up until my grandfather died a few years ago (at 89 himself, I might add)? She worked in the garden most of the year, hoeing, tilling, and picking. Chopping cotton and wood, carrying buckets of coal from the shed to the house, and pumping and toting water from the well in the yard. Chasing kids, grandkids, and great-grandkids – sometimes in play, sometimes with a switch cut from the Rose of Sharon tree in the front yard.

In short, she was active.

And she lived – in great health – to be ninety-three.

July 28

From 1960-1969, fat made up about 40% of the average American's caloric intake. From 1970-1989, it made up about 37%. In the 1990's, it dropped to 33%.

In that same period, obesity in adult America increased by 50%.

Don't believe the hype – if you look closely, even our government will tell you what's most important. Fat isn't what makes you fat; eating too much is what makes you fat.

❧

Today, we had the local homeless shelter come to our house and pick up a whole truckload of stuff we didn't want to take to the new house – a couch, chairs, tons of books, all sorts of things. That's not important, but what *is* important is that I helped load the truck with them. I carried box after box of things down our driveway, single-handedly carried pieces of furniture down stairs and out to the truck, and was able to carry more in a single load than either of the men who came to pick the things up.

Without breaking a sweat.

Later, I went to the U-Haul store to buy some tape and some more boxes. I was carrying all the boxes (20 of them) and the tape to my car in a single load, but dropped the tape midway. Without thinking, I squatted, lowered one end of the box stack to the ground, picked up the tape and put it into my pocket, grabbed the boxes, and stood, taking them the rest of the way to the Jeep without incident.

I tell you these things not to brag, but to share a taste of life as a reasonably fit person, in hopes that you might wish to join me. It's a world of difference on this side of the fence, I can tell you. Surely you don't want me to be alone over here, do you?

Put this book down right now and take a step toward transforming yourself into the person you know you really are. Go for a run. If you cannot run, ride a bike. If you cannot ride a bike, walk. If you cannot walk, find a pool and do some gentle aerobics in the water – that's what I started out doing, back in June of last year. When I started, my exercise was 10 minutes of treading water in the deep end of my pool, because that's all I could do at 371 pounds.

Aren't you worth it?

August 2001

220 – 217 *pounds*

August 5

So here it is, August 5th, 2001. Back in May or June of last year, I decided I would be done dropping my weight by the end of this most recent July.

I'm not done, and I don't care. I fell victim to something most fat people do: I gave myself an unreasonable deadline for dropping almost 200 pounds. We do that, you know. We get excited and motivated, and we decide that we're going to undo the effects of a lifetime of bad living in a week, a month, or a year (depending on just how fat we are).

Sometimes we make it, but more often we don't. We give up, and we get fatter.

So, speaking as someone who's standing closer to end than to the beginning, I'd like to offer up some advice: don't place a burdensome deadline on yourself. Life's too short and too full of other things for that. It's perfectly fine to have a time goal, but the world is not going to end if you miss it. I am proof. (Unless, of course the world's ended and I'm actually in hell now.)

We all have the same destination, and it lies roughly six feet under the surface of the earth. We do not, however, all have the same journey. Instead of aiming for a certain weight by a certain date, why not just aim for improving yourself – your weight, your fitness, your eating choices, your health – just a little bit each and every day? Those tiny improvements start to add up after a while, and before you know it, you're a completely different person.

Enjoy the ride.

August 6

I am.

Those two words are two of the most powerful in the English language. Consider the following:

I am a compulsive overeater.

I am a binger.

I am a fat/carbohydrate/protein/food addict.

I am a big fat pig.

I am out of control.

We use those two words to create labels for ourselves, and by assuming a label, we absolve ourselves of any responsibility for our actions. Labels like the ones above make it easy to eat anything in any quantity, because they give you an excuse. "I couldn't help eating that whole cake," you say, "because I'm a compulsive eater." I know, because I have used that excuse in the past.

Here's an interesting thought: suppose the label you put on yourself influences your actions to support it. I'm not suggesting it's a conscious thing, but what if you tend to binge simply because you tell everyone around you that you're a binger? What if your cravings for candy are increased just because you believe that you are addicted to carbohydrates, because you have been telling yourself that's why you're fat? Is this possible at all?

Labels are very powerful, and the words "I am" are used to create them. Instead of creating labels that limit us and lead to a lack of health, what if we chose to use more empowering ones? What might that do to our health, our opinions of ourselves, and the way we view ourselves? Consider:

I am worth more than any food I eat.

I am a person who loves himself.

I am someone who values her health highly.

I am a person who chooses healthful foods at mealtimes.

I am a thin and fit person.

Believe in yourself and your abilities, and you can make your wildest dreams come true.

August 7

Random thoughts from me to you:

Don't sacrifice your long-term dreams for short-term satisfactions.	If you don't put yourself on a wagon, you cannot fall off one.
You get whatever you settle for.	Aren't you worth more than anything you eat?
If you didn't need a pill to get fat, why would you need one to get unfat?	You can complain about being fat or you can do something about it. Which do you choose?
Live like a thin / fit / healthy person, and you will become one.	The food you eat today dictates the body you have tomorrow.
Keep doing what you've always done and you'll keep getting the results you've always gotten.	Your life is what you choose to make of it, as is your transformation. Would you rather have an easy transformation or a difficult one?
One definition of insanity is: doing the same thing again and again and expecting a different result.	You create your own reality with what you believe. What do you choose to believe about your abilities?
Your past does not equal nor dictate your future.	As much as I hate clichés, nothing does taste as good as fit and healthy feels.
The next year will pass whether you make a decision to change yourself or not.	Don't make any changes to yourself that you are not willing to live with for the rest of your life.
Eat less. Move more.	Don't try. Do.

August 8

Consider the following thoughts of person A:

I am in control.

I can do anything I want to.

I'm going to make transforming into a fit and healthy person the most enjoyable thing I've ever done.

I love myself more than I love food.

Now, contrast those thoughts with these thoughts from person B:

I'm out of control.

I cannot stop myself; I just eat and eat and eat.

Losing this weight is the hardest struggle I've ever been through.

I'm going to cut my calories, but I think I love food too much for it to really work.

Which person would you say has a better chance of transforming from a fat person to a fit person? Your thoughts – your mind – are at the crux of any truly successful change, and those thoughts are entirely under your control.

What do you choose to think?

August 9

I believe I can mentally transform my thoughts in an instant, just by harnessing the power of my mind. I believe I control my every action, and that I choose when, what, and why I eat any food. I believe love for myself is one of the most powerful tools I have. I believe life is all about choices, and that wise choices lead to a healthful life. I believe I am the one who is responsible for me, and I refuse to be anyone's or anything's victim. I believe I am in charge of my eating, not the other way around. I believe I have the power to do anything I set my mind to. I believe you have this same power.

I believe in myself, and I believe in you.

What do you believe?

August 10

I'm a little nervous.

I have to give a presentation next week for work. That doesn't make me nervous; I'm fine with public speaking, as it were, but several of the people who will be present haven't seen me for over a year. That makes me antsy, because I don't really like being the center of attention, and I'm just not looking forward to it.

❧

...take ships as an example. Although they are so large and are driven by strong winds, they are steered by a very small rudder wherever the pilot wants to go. Likewise the tongue is a small part of the body, but it makes great boasts.

Consider what a great forest is set on fire by a small spark. The tongue also is a fire, a world of evil among the parts of the body. It corrupts the whole person, sets the whole course of his life on fire, and is itself set on fire by hell. All kinds of animals, birds, reptiles and creatures of the sea are being tamed and have been tamed by man, but no man can tame the tongue. It is a restless evil, full of deadly poison. (James 3:4-8 NIV)

Strong words, aren't they? They come straight from the Bible, and they're just as timely today as when James penned them almost 2000 years ago. Your tongue, though small, is very powerful, and can direct you much as a rudder steers a ship.

Think about this the next time you:

- Call yourself a "loser," even when talking about weight
- Say you "eat like a pig"
- Tell someone you "hate your body"
- Proclaim that you're "starving to death"
- Label yourself as a food "addict"
- Say that a transformation is a "struggle"
- Tell everyone you're "out of control"

The words you use have power over you. Choose better words, and you can change your attitude and your actions completely.

August 13

What would you do if I told you that all you had to do to transform yourself into the person you desire is to simply start living as though you're already that person? Would you believe in yourself enough to try it, or would you laugh at me and walk away?

I know what it's like to be so fat I couldn't get up from the floor without using a piece of furniture to pull myself up, gasping and red-faced.

I also know what it's like to throw away a bottle of pills I no longer need, and I know what it's like to go run two miles for the hell of it. I've been on both sides of the track, and I have to say, I prefer the side I'm on now.

Know what, though?

I was on this side mentally *long* before I was here physically, and you can be over here with me, if only you allow yourself.

August 16

What do you see when you look in the mirror?

One of the most powerful tools we have is our ability to visualize things that don't exist. Think about how easily you could frighten yourself as a child by simply visualizing a monster under your bed. Myself, I was fond of imagining dead people under there, waiting to reach out and grasp my ankle as I stepped to the floor, and I could work myself into a lather (still can, truth be told) completely by using my imagination.

We can use this same visualization to imagine horrific things – loved ones dying in plane crashes, pets getting hit by cars, children slamming their bikes into trees, and all sorts of gruesome images.

Why waste such a good thing on scaring yourself when you can use it to empower yourself?

Suppose for a moment you decided to harness this power and see a different person when you looked in the mirror each morning? What if, instead of seeing the reality of the fat person you might currently be, you decided to see the person you want to be? What happens then?

See the person you want to be when you look at yourself in the mirror, and it becomes that much easier to eat and live like that person. Eat and live like that person, and I guarantee you'll become that person.

Aristotle said, "We are what we repeatedly do. Excellence then, is not an act, but a habit."

We are what we repeatedly do. Live like the person you want to be, and you'll be that person.

August 18

Who has never used food to avoid something unpleasant? I know I have, and I'm betting most of you have, too. We use food to escape bad feelings from something as simple as an argument with a loved one to something as complex as finding out our child is being disruptive in school. We use food to avoid conflicts so we don't have to deal with the issue at hand.

There are a couple of problems here, though. First, if we don't deal with the conflict, it doesn't go away. It just builds and gets worse. That unresolved argument with the spouse might end in a divorce, and that disruptive child could very well end up in front of a judge in a few years.

And to top it off, you're fat because you put your blinders on and ate your way through it all.

Conflict is an inevitable part of our lives, and we owe it to ourselves to deal with conflicts effectively instead of burying our heads in a pint of Ben and Jerry's. Conflict is not bad. Unpleasant, perhaps, in the short term, but ultimately conflict can be a good thing because we can use it to produce a change, either in ourselves or in someone else. Conflict can also be used to promote unity between people because addressing a conflict allows you to open a line of communication. Talk things through – it can only help.

Don't punish your body out of fear of conflict; you're worth more than that. Face the conflict, resolve it, and grow as a person.

August 20

All too often people "buckle down" and drop some excess weight, get close to a goal they've set, and then suddenly – almost without warning – they seem to reverse direction and end up as big as they were before they started.

Let's look at a typical person, whom I'll call "Bob."

Bob starts shrinking and gets happier and happier. As he becomes the man he wants to be, something happens. An insipid little voice deep down inside him starts whispering to Bob, where no one else can hear.

C'mon, Bob, it says, *you're down over X pounds, lighten up and live a little.*

Bob heeds the voice, and decides to go have that Twinkie that's been on his mind for the last few weeks.

I deserve this, he thinks.

Only he eats the whole box instead of just one. Then, feeling bad about having blown it, he grabs up some Oreos, too, and eats those. Flash ahead a few months, and Bob is rollicking around weighing almost 400 pounds again, and cannot figure out what happened to him.

I know what happened, because it happened to me before.

First, Bob needs to ditch the idea of being "on a diet." Being "on" a diet means you can be "off" a diet.

Second, Bob needs to understand that the occasional Twinkie won't kill him. If he really wants a Twinkie, he should eat a Twinkie. Period. Don't feel like you're forbidden anything – you can eat whatever you choose. If you choose the occasional Twinkie, the world won't end, and it's a whole lot better than depriving yourself until you eat the whole box, right?

Third – and this may be the hardest pill to swallow – if Bob weren't a slave to the scale that little voice in his head might not be so ready to talk. I'd like to take the high road here and act perfect, but the truth is until very recently I was a scale slave too, running to weigh all the time and freaking out if it edged up a pound.

I see things differently now.

My only goal is to continually improve myself, in health and in fitness. I don't have a particular weight goal now like I once did because I've realized there's more to life than what the scales say. If you strive to always make progress in what you're doing with regards to your own body, isn't that a whole lot better than just getting the right number on a scale?

I'd like to invite you to join me in this freedom right now, but I understand if you don't want to yet. It took me over a year to get here, so it would be unreasonable for me to expect anyone to just jump ship with me and see how the water is.

But I'm here when you're ready.

August 21

Comments from me to you:

You *cannot* gain 3, 5, or 10 pounds in a day. Relax, it's probably water.

You *cannot* pack on 5 pounds of muscle a week just from walking. See previous statement.

To become fit, you need a balance of cardio work and resistance (weightlifting) training.

Lifting weights won't make you big and bulky, women readers, because you don't have the testosterone necessary for that.

Fad diets are just that. Fads. Do you still own a pet rock?

For a transformation to be successful, there must be a mental change in the way you view food and eating. Weight loss is merely the physical manifestation of that change.

If a certain food is calling you from the kitchen, either eat it or throw it away. Don't obsess over it.

Although a certain number on the scale may influence how you feel about yourself, it doesn't have to. How you feel is your choice.

You really *do* have enough time to exercise. You're just choosing to make it less important than other things.

If you don't take care of yourself first, how can you take care of those around you?

You can eat whatever you choose. What do you choose to eat?

There are very few foods that are completely unhealthy. Things become unhealthy when we choose to eat these foods in excess.

The less processing that is done to a food, the more of it you can eat, generally. For example, a couple of doughnuts have roughly 610 calories of energy. For that same amount of energy, you can eat a whole pound of shrimp with cocktail sauce, a baked potato with real butter, and a nice big salad. Which do you think would make you feel more satisfied?

You are literally composed of what you consume. Think about that the next time you want one of those doughnuts.

Don't eat for today's pleasure; eat for tomorrow's health.

Dietary fat is not your enemy.

Did you know cocoa powder is one of the best sources of polyphenols (precursors to antioxidants in the blood) there is?

August 28

Tomorrow, I'll make better food choices.
I couldn't hit the gym today, but I'll go later this week.
As soon as I lose a little weight, I'll start exercising.

What do these statements have in common? I know what you're thinking – excuses. But that's not what these are. These are self-promises, and they're the worst kind of promises to break, because when you break them you're simply lying to yourself. I'm pretty good evidence of where a lifetime of broken self-promises get you.

Be true to yourself, you're worth it.

September 2001

September 4

This past Friday I went to a shoe store to get a new pair of running shoes, as I'd discovered a hole in the bottom of the ones I'd been wearing earlier that morning. I used my Visa to pay for the shoes, and the clerk asked me to see some ID since I don't sign the backs of my cards.

We had a short argument because she didn't believe the person in the picture on my driver's license was really me.

❧

Someone asked me today how I feel about fat people, now that I'm no longer one.

Oh boy, what a question. One would probably think – based on some of the things I say in this journal – that I'm now biased against fat people. This is not true. I am, however, more sensitive to the number of fat people there are. It's sort of like you never see someone driving a particular type of vehicle until you buy one. Then they're everywhere.

I feel bad when I see someone as large (or larger) than I once was, because I remember what it's like to be that big. I remember the embarrassment, the stares and laughs, and the physical pain of trying to do simple things like walk up a flight of stairs. I remember complaining every four to six weeks to my also-large wife about how we needed to "do something" about our weight, and I also remember not doing anything about it.

I remember all this, and it hurts to see people who are where I was. Hurts to see the unhappy faces, hurts to watch them sitting and resting because a short walk tired them out, hurts to witness someone walking out of an amusement park ride because she didn't fit in the seat. It hurts because there's so much more to life than just sitting back and watching it pass you by.

It hurts knowing that no matter how much I want to walk up to those people and say "I can help you," I cannot walk up to them and say that, because I remember how many times people tried to help me in the past to no avail. I simply ended up feeling bad about myself. We all have to make our choices in this life, and we all have to live with the results of those choices. It sounds rough, but it's a true statement.

Hopefully this book will help some of those people, even though I'm well aware that many times I say things that cause pain, maybe even seem hateful and biased. They're not intended to be, but the truth does sometimes sound harsh and I don't apologize for that.

September 5

You can get a better cardio workout on a bicycle if you keep it in a lower gear and pedal faster. This works out particularly well if you're one of those people who do their cardio in the dark, as I tend to be. It's also a lot easier to see pedestrians when you're only going ten miles per hour.

September 6

I have the holy shits.

No, they're not some sort of charismatic diarrhea, they're small bullets of time when it hits me – all of the sudden – just how much different I am now, as opposed to pre-May 2000. I'll be minding my own business, doing something at work, perhaps, or sitting in front of the TV, and it dawns on me: I'm a whole new man these days.

And I think, *holy shit!*

Why? Because it fills me with surprise every time it happens, a sense of wonder at the path my life's taken, and it simply amazes me. I get totally stunned – and I don't know how well I'll be able to put it into words here – because I'm suddenly aware that I'm not the big fat blob of a man I was, that sometime over the last few months the visualized Fred from the mirror stepped out and took his place, and I feel like I wasn't even aware of it. It's like I was fat, then suddenly I was not fat.

First comes surprise and amazement, then gratitude. Gratitude that I'm living now, instead of dying. Gratitude that I no longer have diabetes – that, in fact, the only problems I have with my health now are injuries caused by being too *active*, rather than too fat and sedentary. Gratitude that I finally woke up and smelled the proverbial coffee.

Generally, a "thank God" moment follows closely behind a holy shit.

September 9

Losing weight is really a matter of simple physics, even if it's an unpopular belief. The equation can be summed up in this statement:

If you consume fewer calories than you expend, you will lose weight.

Some people lose weight more slowly because of a few reasons:

They have less lean (muscle) mass. This is far and away the biggest reason for the "men lose faster than women" comment I hear all the time. Since men have more muscle, and muscle is an active tissue – meaning it requires energy even at rest – men require more calories daily.

The energy you expend when you do cardio work is related to two things: intensity and duration. I hate to say this, because it's going to piss off a lot of people, but a slow leisurely stroll doesn't cut the mustard for most people (super-sized people are different with regards to this). If you want to elevate your metabolism, you have to get your heart rate hiked up. Most experts recommend getting your heart rate up to 60%-80% of its maximum rate for optimal benefits.

Many people want to only do cardio work (I myself was guilty of this), not taking into account the benefits of resistance training. Numerous studies show that resistance training elevates the metabolism for up to 24 hours following an intense workout, compared to about a one-hour elevation after a cardio workout. Then there's the whole idea that a single pound of muscle burns up to 50 calories a day all by itself, which also elevates the metabolism.

It's possible that the "yo-yo dieter" theory holds a little validity, though I have yet to read a single study that supports the idea. The theory is as follows: a person loses weight rapidly on some fad diet, and ultimately loses more muscle than fat. They then go off the diet and gain their weight (and more, in all likelihood) back. The weight they regain, according to the theory, is fat, and their resting metabolism gets slower and slower because each time this happens they have less muscle mass.

I've read of one study that actually contradicts the yo-yo dieter theory. The study showed that as a person gained weight, they gained enough muscle to allow their body to carry around the additional fat, which appears to discount the theory.

Eat less. Move more. It really works.

September 15

It was nice this morning, walk-jogging in the September cool. I found something out fast, though.

Fifty-seven degrees when you weigh in the low 200's feels a lot different than when you weigh in the upper 300's. I nearly froze to death.

September 17

I now weigh less than 20 pounds more than I did at my high school graduation, and I'm in damn better shape.

You cannot control external events in your life. You never know when tragedy or hardship may strike, and you don't know when life's going to be the proverbial bowl of cherries. Certain things are out of our control. Our responses to those events are, however, entirely in our control. How you choose to react to any given situation lies completely within your grasp.

You're in complete control of what you put in your mouth, no matter what's going on in the world. You're also in control of your activity choices.

Being in control is a good thing, because it gives us power in times when we may feel powerless. No matter what happens to me, be it a tragic event, a vacation, or anything, I rest better knowing that I'm still in charge of myself, and will continue to be in charge.

September 21

If you put a PowerBar in the fridge, don't use the microwave to try and soften it, unless you've got some extra skin on the roof of your mouth that you don't need.

Just so you know, of course, because I'd never actually do anything so dumb.

September 22

You know your life has really changed when you start looking for exercise-type-things to do when you get bored.

September 24

Are you watching life pass you by while you sit on the sidelines, getting fatter and fatter?

Why?

Aren't you worth more than that?

You only get one shot at life, and then you die. The choices you make today have a direct impact on the quality of the life you have tomorrow. Choose poorly today, and you get rewarded with heart disease, diabetes, atherosclerosis, and an early death. Choose wisely, however, and you greatly reduce your chances of having any of those problems. Matter of fact, if you already have some of them, wise choices with regards to food and physical activity can even reverse the effects.

What sort of life do you want?

September 25

- Diabetes.
- Heart disease.
- Cancer: breast, ovarian, uterine, esophageal, colorectal, renal cell, and prostate.
- Hypertension. Pancreatitis. Impaired respiratory functions.
- Pregnancy complications. Birth defects.
- Stroke. Sleep apnea. Acid reflux disease.
- Infertility. Gallstones. Impaired immune response.
- Osteoarthritis. Rheumatoid arthritis. Infections.

- Gynecological disorders. Obesity hypoventilation syndrome.
- Liver disease. Hyperlipidemia. Atherosclerosis.
- Impotence. Carpal tunnel syndrome. Chronic venous insufficiency.
- Deep vein thrombosis. End stage renal disease.
- Incontinence.
- Gallbladder disease. Abdominal hernias.
- Hypoxia. Gout. Low back pain.

What do they all have in common? They're complications of obesity. Is that what you want out of life? The choices are yours, every single day. Will you live for the taste today, or for the health tomorrow?

October 2001

211 – 209 *pounds*

October 1

Everyone knows that aerobic exercise – cardio, to you and me – burns up calories and body fat while you're doing it, and even keeps burning them for a while after you quit.

That's pretty cool.

Lifting weights, however, boosts your metabolism for 24 hours or more after you do it intensely – even when you're sleeping. You're burning all sorts of energy while your body is recovering and rebuilding the muscle tissue you worked.

Some other nifty weightlifting factoids you might not know:

- Weight training can reverse the natural decline in your metabolism that starts about age 30.
- It lowers your chances of getting adult-onset diabetes.
- It lowers your blood pressure and your resting heart rate.
- It improves your coordination (something I desperately need) and your posture.
- It speeds the transit of materials through your digestive tract, thus lowering your risks of colon or rectal cancer.
- It improves your immune system and your endurance.
- It can prevent or reverse osteoporosis.
- It increases the HDL (good) cholesterol in your blood.
- It elevates your mood and gives you more energy.

Are you lifting weights yet?

October 6

Someone asked me today how Robyn and I get Danielle to eat healthy foods. We generally don't have trouble with her, because we don't keep much junk food around the house. She snacks on unsweetened applesauce and yogurt, mostly. I'm a big believer in the "if they're hungry, they'll eat it" school of thought when it comes to healthful foods, for the very most part.

I don't mean that in an abusive way – we'd never force her to eat something she absolutely cannot stand, like meatloaf. She gets options for things like that. Most of the time however, it's not a matter of disliking a particular food, it's a matter of wanting a crappy food more. If there's no choice, though, it's amazing what a child will eat.

Something that Robyn and I find helpful with our daughter is discussing various foods with her, and how they affect the human body when consumed. I mean things like:

"This salmon is very good for you because it's one of the best sources we have for a special fat our brains need."

"This bread has lots of fiber in it, which helps you poop good (Danielle and I love our poop talks). That white bread doesn't have any poop-helper in it."

"These cookies aren't so good for you because they have a lot of sugar."

You get the idea. We explain things to her more or less on her level, and she seems to be getting a decent understanding of what's good for her and what's not. She tells us regularly about how she could've had a big piece of cake at school but she had a small one instead, or how she had a salad instead of a second cookie.

One thing we try to impress upon her is that most things aren't too terribly unhealthy, as long as she doesn't have too much of them.

"Fred," she asks often, "is _______ bad for you?"

My response is generally something like, "________ is not terribly bad, but *too much* _______ is bad for you." I make sure to point out that it's entirely possible to even have too much of a good thing.

The one thing that's particularly helpful is the fact that Robyn and I were once both super-sized, and Danielle remembers how we never did anything but sit around and eat. She sees us moving around now, doing things, and she knows about how I don't need to take pills any more and how we're never sick like we used to be. Being a living example to her of what bad health is like versus what good health is like, and all that.

Teach your kids, but don't lecture them. And remember, they'll follow your example, and they'll learn from your attitude. If you bitch and moan about losing weight, and how "hard" it is to eat right, that will rub off on them. Show them just how much more fun it is to be healthy and in good shape.

October 11

Last night, as I lay in bed tossing and turning, trying to sleep, I had an idea I'd like to mention. I spend a great deal of time preaching the good news of health and fitness, but I don't ever really touch on a couple of the negative sides to having dropped a lot of weight. I'm not talking about expected negatives, like loose skin, I'm talking about the ones I never saw coming.

Interjection: There is no way these negatives even come close to the positives, so don't think I'm trying to tell you making the commitment to change yourself isn't worth it. It is worth it, every little bit. For every negative there are at least a hundred positives. These are just things I didn't anticipate at the beginning.

I never imagined I would be so damn cold. At 371 pounds, the house was 68 degrees all the time, and I still managed to sweat considerably. Now we keep it around 75 or 77, and my teeth chatter.

When I was super-fat, I wore shorts through the winter and made fun of all the skinny people who said, "Aren't you cold?" Smugly (I have a history of smugness) I'd reply, "Cold is just a state of mind."

I was an idiot.

Now I stand around shivering and wonder how all the skinny people can sit in the office in mere shirtsleeves, or I crank the heat up so much people bitch at me.

I also never dreamed I'd bruise so easily. I always have a bruise here or there, it seems. Most of them come from the trials of being active but I have a set of almost constant bruises on the inside of each leg, just below the knee. These spots on my legs are literally more often bruised than not. Know why?

Because my big bony knees bang together at night when I'm in bed.

There's no padding there any more, just skin and bone around my knees, and the clacking together during the night keeps me bruised on both legs. I've actually started sleeping with a pillow between my knees to prevent it.

Once again, I've managed to make myself sound like a freak.

October 13

I was reflecting in the shower this morning, as I often do, thinking about how my thinking has changed over the last 17 months.

Back at the beginning, I was obsessed with how much I weighed. Now I don't really care much at all. I check my weight regularly still, but without the trepidation I once had. If it goes up, it goes up; if it goes down, it goes down. As long as I'm working toward improving my health and fitness, I'm going the right way.

My idea of what I needed to eat then was way different from now. Then, it worked out to about 1800 calories a day, in three big meals. Now it's closer to 3000 calories a day, in five or six smaller meals. I cannot help but laugh when I think back to the day about six months ago when I first tried eating six meals and stopped after a single day because it was such a pain in the butt. Now I don't see how I ever got by just eating three times a day.

At the beginning, I didn't care so much for what I was eating – except for sugar – but I cared how much of it I was eating. Now I care *far* more about what it is I'm putting in my mouth than how much of it I'm putting in. For example: we used to eat out more, and I'd just eat less fast food. Now I pretty much don't eat fast food at all, because I know what it's doing inside my body.

Then, all I did was cardio work, because I thought I was "too fat" to lift weights. Now, weightlifting is a huge part of my fitness training. You're never too fat to start training with weights. Weights are far too good for you to ever ignore. When I started training with weights, I thought machines were the best things ever. Now I think a good balance of free weights and machines are optimal.

October 14

Someone recently asked me if I regret having been fat, or if I'm glad I walked in a fat man's shoes.

I have mixed emotions. When I was merely portly, say, up to about 260 or 270 pounds, I was the proverbial life of the party. I was happy-go-lucky, loud, obnoxious and an all-around fun guy. I had an understanding that I was fat, but it didn't seem to bother anyone, and it didn't really bother me. I don't regret this time at all.

Then I crossed the 300-pound mark, and things changed.

I became quiet, withdrawn, and embarrassed to be seen by people. I stopped going into public except when it was absolutely necessary, and I stopped going to family functions, including weddings and funerals. I let my friends fall by the wayside, one by one. Soon, the only friends I had outside of work "friends" were all online, because that's where I spent most of my time.

When you're online, no one knows how fat you are.

By the time I crossed 350 pounds, Robyn and I were having our groceries delivered so we didn't have to go to the store. We didn't go anywhere together, because it embarrassed me too much. A super-fat person in public is bad enough (my thinking at the time went), but two super-fatties together draw so much attention it's unbearable. I had (and still have, at times) tendencies to care a little too much what people think about me.

As a result of these things, I missed a good six or seven years of living my life, and I regret the hell out of that. I regret the damage I've done to my body because I didn't care enough to take care of it. I regret driving away all my friends, and I regret alienating large sections of my family.

Qualifier for the previous paragraph: I met my wife – the best thing that's ever happened to me – during that time. When I refer to "missing out on living," I'm talking about doing things: going places without shame, participating in living, enjoying things life had to offer. Stuff like that.

All I can these days is make up for lost time, which I'm doing every single day. Things are healed with the family, but I still have no friends.

This would be a good reason to join a gym, I'm thinking.

The good thing about having been so fat is that I can now speak definitively about it, from experience. I know how it feels to be laughed at, to be sick all the time, to have trouble walking, and that gives me the ability to empathize with fat people I encounter. It also gives me compassion towards them, even if I sometimes sound like I don't have it when I'm writing. For that I'm grateful.

See what I mean about mixed emotions? Yes I regret having been fat because I feel like I missed several fun years, but now that I'm not fat I'm glad I have the perspective on life that I have.

I've seen both sides, and I must say, this side is much more enjoyable.

October 17

I had to go to a customer's site today, and because it is a government facility I had to wear a badge and get escorted back to the area where the people I was meeting were. The guy that came out to escort me did a slight double take when he saw me, but he didn't say anything. I'm betting he thought I had cancer, or something. God knows I've heard that one before. Cancer, or AIDS.

We walked back to the meeting area, and I saw all the people I hadn't seen for well over a year. No one mentioned anything about me looking remotely different – not even mentioning the fact that I'm wearing contacts now instead of glasses.

The conversation went on, and we were working out a particular problem when one of the women and I had a minor disagreement on how some software I wrote a couple of years back worked.

"It won't work on Windows NT at all," she said, slightly belligerently.

"Yes it does," I said, "There are 64 other sites who'd beg to differ with you."

"It does not," she replied, "the guy who originally worked on it came over here and tried. His name was..."

She scrunched up her face, deep in thought. The rest of us waited.

"I think *his* name was Fred, too, now that I think about it," she finished.

At that point, hilarity ensued.

October 20

I just finished digging a daffodil bed for Robyn (she'll be doing the actual planting, I was just the laborer). I learned a couple of things.

At 210-ish pounds, it's a whole lot easier to dig a flowerbed than in was when I was in the 370's. I barely broke a sweat. However, I cannot drive the shovel nearly as deep when I'm breaking the ground. I'm sure I looked quite the fool out there, jumping up and down on the shovel.

But I'm used to that.

What kind of person do you want to be? Do you have a vision for that? All too often, people get caught up in the idea of simply "losing weight," and don't get a vision for what they want to be. If you have a vision, you can accomplish anything you want.

I have a vision. Every time I look in the mirror I see it – that man I want to be. I saw him then, and I see him now. He once existed only in my head, now he's mostly real. He's not completely here yet, but he's much, *much* closer, just under the surface.

Do you have a vision for the person you want to be? If you have a vision, you have something concrete to look forward to. Without a vision, you're destined to fall, and the landing hurts like hell.

October 21

A sign you've transformed: you find yourself now concerned with how loose your clothes are, rather than how tight they are.

Sometimes I feel sorry for the people who have to put up with me. Take that poor cashier at the grocery store yesterday, for example, when I was loading my groceries on the conveyor.

"Did you get any Italian bread?" she asked, perkily, while she scanned my items.

"No, I didn't," I replied, laying my organic brown eggs on the belt.

"It's on sale right now for fifty..."

"Sorry, I don't eat white bread," I interrupted. Then, feeling like I'd sounded rude, I added, "But that sounds like a great price."

"It's a great price," she said.

She scanned another couple of items then tried a different tack.

"What about vitamin C? It's only ninety-nine cents!"

"No thanks, I get all the vitamins I need from the foods I eat."

Her face fell, and she didn't speak again until I'd completely emptied my cart. She tried a third line, which I guess was based on my responses to her previous questions.

"My sister," she said as she scanned my organic salad mix, "is trying that Atkins Diet, where they can't have any carbohydrates, and she can't eat any salad. I didn't know salad was considered a complex carbohydrate."

"I didn't know that, either," I concurred.

"She can eat all the meat she wants: pork, beef, whatever. But no breads, no potatoes, nothing like that."

"It's amazing, isn't it," I said, "The crazy things people will do to lose weight? They'll eat any weird food, try any funky fad diet, or take any pill, but they won't do the common sense thing and just eat healthier foods and move their butts a little bit."

She agreed, and I think she was happy to finally find something we could talk about, because she went on to tell me about how she'd dropped 27 pounds with Weight Watchers a couple of years ago, but had put the weight right back on when she stopped going to the meetings.

The last thing she told me before I left was that she needed to sign back up.

October 22

Nothing stings quite like a resistance band breaking right in the middle of a full outer thigh stretch, when you've got it looped around both legs.

At least this week I'll know for sure where those bruises came from.

October 23

From time to time, I see things happen that hit a resonant chord within me. One such incident happened today.

Each morning before I get ready for work, the first thing I do is give our cats plenty of food. Without fail, our cat, Snoopy, waits for me, and eats like a condemned man getting his last meal.

Today was no different. He ate while I peed. He ate while I brushed my teeth. He was still eating when I got out of the shower. He attacked the food like he was a cop and the 9-lives was a box of doughnuts.

While I was combing my hair it happened. Snoopy made a series of nasty retching sounds, and proceeded to lay an 8-inch vomit log, solid and made of cat food, in the bowl and on top of the remaining food. He sat back and licked his lips a few times, then looked up at me.

"Snoopy, that's nasty!" I proclaimed from my vantage point by the sink.

I dried my hands and walked over to where he sat, picked up the bowl, and just dumped everything in the toilet. Snoopy meowed bitchily at me, as is his way.

I refilled the food bowl and put it in its spot by the water bowl, then returned to combing my hair at the sink. Within 30 seconds, he had his face back in the bowl, grunting and crunching. I just watched him eat.

That was me, I thought, *eighteen months ago.* I didn't have bulimia, don't get me wrong here, but I did the fat person equivalent to what he was doing. I would eat, and eat, and eat, until I felt sick to my stomach. Not puking sick, but nauseated sick. I'd eat until I couldn't stand it, then I'd go sit on the couch and complain about being so full.

For about a half hour. Then I was back in the kitchen eating a little of this, tasting a little of that. I'd like to take the easy way out here and claim that I was "compulsive," or "obsessed," like I hear others do – hell, if you'd asked me then I'd have probably used that excuse – but the truth is far less complex and not nearly as pretty.

The truth is, I loved food, and that's no excuse at all. When it came to eating, I made poor choices, based on taste and convenience, and not at all on knowledge, and I ate my way up to almost 400 pounds.

I still love food, but food serves a different purpose now. Food, I've realized, is literally what composes my body. You are what you eat, and I don't like the body that the Big Mac built.

What's building your body?

October 26

Some scientists now blame obesity on a certain gene that prevents our bodies from effectively using the protein leptin, thus making us fat. What a load of baloney.

The human genetic code did *not* magically change to suddenly make over 60% of American adults fat in the last generation. We're fat because we eat too much garbage – not too much quantity, necessarily, but too much garbage with no nutritional value – and we eat it in the middle of a day of sitting on our wide butts. We're fat, yet we're starving to death because we're not giving our bodies the nutrition they need.

That's why.

I don't know any plainer way to state it than that. I know some of you reading this probably disagree with me, and I know that we're all different. I'm not trying to make a "one size fits all" argument.

I will say this, though: I believe one size fits most.

Losing weight, being healthy, whatever you choose to call it, is pretty simple, no matter what the people who want to sell you something will try to tell you. It's about how you decide to live, what you decide to eat, and how willing you are to take full responsibility for your actions.

October 27

Yesterday, I wrote that most people were fat because they ate a lot of garbage foods with no nutritional value. Empty calories, so to speak. I'm sure you've heard the phrase. I commented that people didn't "necessarily" eat too much food, just too much nutritionally void food.

I wrote that before we took Danielle to dinner for her birthday last night. She ordered grilled chicken, fries, and a side salad and Robyn and I decided to split a steak because we knew that it would be too much for one of us. We all ordered Bleu Cheese salad dressing on the side for our salads – Robyn and I because we know that restaurants tend to float the salads in dressing otherwise, and Danielle because she just wanted to do what we were doing.

Our salads came, and the little side-servings of dressing were easily a half-cup each. That's about eight times what I normally put on a salad *bigger* than the one they served me – and the salads I make don't have the generous half-cup of cheddar cheese dumped on top, either.

When the main course was served, the steak was nearly an inch thick and covered more than half of the oversized plate. Our potato was small, and they'd tried to get us to order it with butter, sour cream, bacon, and cheese. Danielle received two entire chicken breasts, a huge pile of thick cut steak fries, and a half-cup of honey mustard dressing. It appeared that both our steak and her chicken had been basted with oil or butter while they were cooking, because they were both sitting in big pools of grease.

Is it any wonder we're the fattest nation on earth?

Don't blame the restaurants, though. They're just serving us what we want, and like good little boys and girls we make every effort to clean our plates. We've lost sight of what a normal serving is – believe it or not, the steak that Robyn and I shared was four servings – and we Americans are eating our way into the record books.

I'm not advocating avoiding eating out, and I'm not advocating boycotting restaurants. What I am advocating is that we start paying attention to what we're putting into our bodies. There's no rule anywhere that says you have to clean your plate at a restaurant, and there's nothing that says you cannot have control over how your food is prepared.

Don't eat, then regret. Think before you eat.

October 28

Yesterday, I decided to drive over to the river with Danielle, to a spot where I once fished regularly, both in my childhood and during my college years. We walked around for a bit when we got there, balancing on the railroad tracks that run along the river's edge and throwing rocks into the water. As we turned to head back to the car, I saw it: a playground, with no one in it at all.

So we played, and I discovered something I never knew. Playgrounds are easily as much fun, if not *more* fun, when you're an adult. Jungle gyms. Monkey bars. Seesaws. Merry-go-rounds. Slides – head first, feet first, and butt first. They were all simply incredible. Incredible, yes, but there was something far more than just incredible. There were swings.

I can play on the swings again. My butt fits just fine in the seats, and there's no fear of breaking the chains ever again. But the feeling, oh my God, the feeling of the wind in your face, of seeing the ground race toward you and then the swoosh and suddenly you're rocketing into the blue sky, grinning like a hound dog hanging out a truck window on the highway because you cannot *not* grin, reaching the apex pumping your legs and struggling to overcome the urge to jump out of the seat and pretend you're a paratrooper, and then you're headed toward the ground again only this time you're going backwards and there's another swoosh and at the bottom you kick at the ground so you'll go just a little higher, and then you're moving up now watching the ground diminish below you, and you realize your head's going higher than the top bar of the swing set and you idly wonder if you could loop-the-loop and then there's a pause, and the chain goes slack in your hand and for one sickening moment your stomach rushes into your throat and then you repeat the whole process over and over and over.

October 29

For the record: if you find yourself on a swing set, swinging high, and get the sudden urge to leap from your seat like you're a kid, keep in mind that your adult weight will cause you to hit the ground with a far greater force than your youthful weight did.

I'm pretty sure the bruise on the inside of my foot will fade in a few days.

October 30

Hey, hey, according to the "fun facts" page on the National Soft Drink Association's web site, Americans consumed more than 53 gallons of soft drink per person in 2000.

Fifty-three gallons. Per person.

Have a Coke and a smile.

November 2001

210 – 206 *pounds*

November 1

In America, we'll wait three hours in line for a sugar coated and deep fried doughnut when a new Krispy Kreme is opening, and then wonder why we're so fat.

Must be genetics, we say, *I've got that damn obesity gene.*

It's just my set point, my body won't let me be a healthy size, we tell our friends.

I barely eat anything at all, we cry, *I think I'm just destined to be fat.*

We make excuses, and we refuse to be responsible for our actions. I'll let you in on a little secret, my friends. Responsibility is power. When you decide to take responsibility for your actions – and your weight and health – you become the master of your own destiny. You can guide, or you can be guided.

Who's running your life?

November 2

I'd like to pose a few questions to those who are unhappy with your weight and fitness level, if I may.

That Whopper you had for lunch today, was it worth it?

Was skipping that workout on Wednesday morning worth it?

What about the Snickers bar you snuck out of your kid's Halloween candy? (You didn't think I knew about that one, did you?) Was it worth it?

And you – you know who you are – the one who snuck a Reese's cup out of the Halloween candy for yourself every time you handed one out, were those worth it?

Are you ready for the curve now? I think in many cases they *were* worth it. Worth every little bite, every extra ten minutes in bed.

Here's the problem, though: we tend to let those things snowball on us, and we're very good at forgetting our past. When we eat the Whopper on Friday, we've forgotten all about sneaking the Snickers bar Thursday while the kid was at school. While we're digging that Snickers bar out, we're not mindful of all the Reese's cups we grabbed out of the big bowl by the door the night before. Of course, as we're eating those Reese's cups, we've long since forgotten tapping the snooze button that morning to skip the workout.

That, friends, is what makes you become a behemoth 371-pound man who does nothing but sit around, eat, and complain about being so fat. No single incident can do that; it takes a lot of incidents, and they add up. Then you pay for them in spades, with an early death from complications of some obesity-related disease or being homebound because you cannot get around any more.

The moral? Enjoy the Snickers. Skip a workout. Have a Whopper.

But think first. Engage your mind before you engage your mouth. Like I said, an incident is not a problem; that doesn't happen until it becomes a pattern.

November 3

I talk with people regularly who are "trying to lose weight." Lots of people, and many have one thing in common. I've been guilty of this before, so don't think I'm looking down from some high vantage point here. I've been there.

The thing they have in common is starvation.

Not the mental one, where you think, "I'm starving" all the time because you're hungry, but a literal one. The absolute minimum energy a human needs to survive is (I know there are many factors affecting these numbers, like age, weight, climate, and health; I'm generalizing again) 1200 calories a day for women and 1500 calories a day for men.

That's what you need to stay alive. Barely. Problem is, when you cut yourself back to the bare minimum, several things happen: your body's survival mechanism kicks in, and you begin to cannibalize your lean tissue (muscle). Since your body's in starvation mode, it takes the path of least resistance. Protein (muscle) is easier to utilize than fat is (because fat's a more complex structure), so say goodbye to a few pounds of muscle. You drop a few pounds of muscle and water weight then stick at a certain point on the scale. It's not a set point, like some want you to think, it's the point where your body – realizing you're starving to death – starts conserving every little bit of energy you consume, because your system thinks there's a famine.

Often, people start to gain weight at this point, for a couple of reasons. One, your body's conserving everything you ingest, because it's a very efficient machine, and two, since you've lost some muscle mass, you need less energy to survive (i.e., you have a lower metabolic rate), and therefore more energy can be stored as fat.

You get disgusted with this crappy, overly restrictive starvation diet, and start eating normally again. You pick your water weight back up, and since your metabolic rate is slower right now, you probably pick up a little fat, too. Contrary to popular belief, however, that muscle mass will come back. No matter what the diet gurus who want your money tell you, you cannot yo-yo diet yourself into being permanently fat. The muscle comes back because your body needs it to support your new fat.

So you end up fatter after your "diet" than you were before you started. The one other time I made a semi-serious attempt to "lose weight" I weighed 330 pounds at the beginning. I started eating between 1000-1200 calories a day, and dropped almost 50 pounds in about three months. And stalled. And gave up. And weighed 371 pounds before I knew it.

Most women need in the neighborhood of 1700-2200 calories a day to be healthy, and most men need somewhere around 2500-3500. Again, these numbers are generalized – active men in cold climates may need 7000 or more calories a day to be healthy – and there are always exceptions to my generalizations.

Don't be stupid. Don't starve yourself. If you simply start eating the foods your body was designed to eat in reasonable quantities, and moving your butt in activities you enjoy, true miracles can, and will, happen. Fat will melt away. Blood pressure will go down. Chronic diseases like diabetes, in my case, may vanish. Your clothes get baggy, and people around you start to tell you how good you're looking.

November 7

From all my chatting with people who want to "lose weight," I've noticed something peculiar. Without fail, those of us who've dropped semi-large amounts of weight all have something in common: we've all basically modified the quantity and quality of what we eat, and we've become more active than we once were. We've then proceeded to habitually do these things.

Interestingly enough, we're the ones that most people are unwilling to listen to. They want to know about the cabbage soup diet, or the Atkins diet, or Meridia, or weight-loss surgery, or anything except the way to actually succeed.

Why is that?

We're a sensible people for the most part, reasonable, except about one thing: our health. We abuse our bodies year after year, getting fatter and fatter and picking up complication after complication, until we reach some point where we feel like we have to change.

And we lose our minds.

We try to undo 20 (or more) years of unhealthy living by spending a few days having a "juice fast" to "remove the toxins" from our bodies. We wire our jaws shut, or have pretty much our entire stomach removed. We buy a pill that makes us crap out excess fat or one that hypes up our heart rate so high it could possibly be dangerous. We drink our green tea, because we heard that it's a "natural metabolism booster," and we consume mass quantities of any supplement we think might help us get to some magical scale number.

Be sensible. It took time to get fat; take a little time to get not-fat. I remember how it felt to be that big, but I also remember how it felt to fail at the fads time and time again. Take your time, enjoy the process, and watch the miracle unfold before your eyes. You're worth the wait.

November 10

I witnessed something interesting a couple of days ago. I had the opportunity to watch a very large (350-400 pounds) woman lecture someone on the dangers of smoking, while punctuating her argument with bites from a giant Twizzler stick.

This, friends, is the word "denial" in action.

We get one shot at life, and only one. If you feel like you've screwed your life up, take heart: you can change things right now, if only you want to. All it takes is a single decision followed by some action, and it's as easy as you choose for it to be. You can change your life for the better right now, if only you want to, or you can take the alternative route and live in denial: eating everything in sight and sitting on your ass all day and pretending that your knees really don't hurt that bad or that the pounding of your heart after walking across a room is normal or that you didn't really want to ride roller coasters ever again or that people aren't really staring at you or that you don't really mind getting all your clothes at special stores.

Really, it's easy to do if you try.

Just shut yourself off from the world and create the reality you want. Remember, that's always an alternative, because we create our own realities. Just pretend you're not hurting, pretend you don't see the looks or hear the comments, pretend you don't mind the thoughts that you'll die young, and you'll be just fine. Me, I'll take the better way. I've tried both and I've found that I love running and playing and swinging and fitting and climbing and wrestling and moving and living far too much to ever go back to that other place.

Imagine a world where you can buy clothes anywhere; where you can do anything you want; where you're the person outside that you always knew about inside. That world is yours for the taking, if only you'll let yourself reach out and take it.

If only.

November 11

For the last several days, I've been slopping lotion all over my hands several times a day, trying to fix what I thought was the worst case of dry skin I've ever had. Last night, I figured out what it is.

I have calluses all over my hands from lifting weights. Turns out Robyn has them, too, but she's known what hers were from day one.

Sometimes I think I'm just a little on the slow side. I *am* from Alabama, you know.

November 15

Can you imagine what it would feel like to be five years younger? Ten? Twenty?

Can you imagine having boundless energy to do anything you want to?

Can you imagine not being ashamed to look at yourself in the mirror?

You can have everything you can imagine, if you want to. This is not an infomercial, and I'm not going to make you any promises about how you can transform yourself in just minutes a day. I will tell you this, however: if you can dream it, you can make it happen.

If you want it.

Would you like to be able to pick things up off the floor without your face turning red and your pulse jumping up? Would you like to be able to fit in normal chairs and shop in normal stores? Would you like to be seated at a booth in a restaurant without worrying about whether you'll have to move the table or request a non-booth seat?

I wished for those things too, for many years, so I know how it feels. I know the pain, and I know the emotional hurt – even if I sound like I've forgotten it sometimes. I also know the secret to making all those dreams come true. I can sum it up in one word, if you like.

Love. That's all it takes. Love yourself.

Loving yourself is easy, contrary to what you might think. It's not emotional, and it's not mystical. Like so many other things in this life, it's a choice. You can choose to love yourself, no matter how long you've hated yourself. You can choose to let go of all your old pains and frustrations, and simply start loving you for what you are. Go ahead, you're worth it. Give it a try.

With love comes the realization that you're not treating yourself with love. Love doesn't make you eat until you're ready to vomit – and then want to eat some more. Love doesn't keep your butt in the chair in front of the television. Love moves you, and it shows you that you're far more valuable than any piece of food.

Love yourself, and make your dreams come true. Can you imagine?

November 19

For the record: it is my carefully considered opinion that natural peanut butter and homemade strawberry jam on whole wheat bread is about the best snack ever, especially when it's right between lunch and dinner and you're hungry.

November 21

If any of you are coming to the Huntsville area for Thanksgiving and happen to find a testicle on the side of the road while here, it's mine. I lost one this morning while running. Please keep it warm, and send it to me.

I had no idea the low 20's would feel so cold. Go figure. Take away almost half the man and his tolerance changes drastically. I was even wearing full sweats, gloves, and I had the hood of my sweatshirt up.

All that, and one still broke off, rolled down my leg and I never found it in the dark.

Fortunately I went to the store today, and bought additional gloves, thermal underwear (top and bottom), thicker socks, and a little wool cap to wear on my head.

Hopefully I can make it through tomorrow's walk-jog without losing the other one.

November 23

One of the most heartbreaking things I can imagine is to be on my deathbed and to have regrets for all the things I never did because I was too fat. Really, who wants to do that? I missed a goodly chunk of my youth – my twenties – because I was too fat, and I'm doing my best to make up for that now. That's why I'm doing things like playing in the park, throwing footballs, and riding my daughter's scooter.

I could not, and then I could. And can. And do.

I would wager that for the vast majority of my large readers, it's not too late to recapture some of that lost youth, if only you want to. Do you want to? Nothing makes you feel quite as free as playing like a kid again

– you forget all about the troubles that life hands you. That freedom is yours for the taking if you want it. I know how the freedom feels, as does my wife. We know the feeling of freedom – freedom from being tired all the time, freedom from health problems caused by obesity, freedom from the Sword-of-Damocles threat of an early death due to complications from obesity.

Most of all, we know the feeling of freedom that comes from being able to do anything we want, and I'd be willing to bet that none of us will ever be going back to where we were.

Won't you join us? All it takes is a single decision to change.

November 24

Yesterday I called a local day spa and made an appointment for a 1:45 massage, my first ever. I was nervous about disrobing in front of a strange woman, but she was very good at putting me at ease. She let me leave my underwear on, which made me practically comfortable. The massage was an hour, and she did several different styles. All was well until she started working on my legs. On my thighs, actually.

And I popped wood – the kind a cat couldn't scratch – right there in her face.

I was mortified, to put it lightly. My mind went blank as I desperately tried to think of something – *anything* – to say.

"Heh," I tried, smiling weakly at her.

"Hmm?" she asked, looking up at me.

I looked at my crotch, then back at her.

"I guess I'm enjoying this a little more than I thought I was," I said, my face flaring a bright red.

"Pardon?" she asked.

I nodded my head in the erection direction.

"I guess I'm enjoying this a little more than I thought I was," I repeated, praying for the ground to open up and swallow me.

"Oh, that," she said, "That happens all the time. I didn't even notice."

She didn't even notice.

Dissed by the massage lady.

November 25

While I'm thinking about it – this is related to my day-spa story from yesterday – I'm insanely ticklish, to the point of embarrassment should anyone ever see or hear me when I get tickled, and I had zero problems at the day spa. No little girly giggles, no high-pitched screeches, and no jumping around like a Mexican jumping bean.

There was one frightening moment when she was working between my toes during the pedicure, but I maintained my composure.

I give you this information should you also be very ticklish, to let you know they use a very firm touch, and don't tickle you at all.

You're on your own with your erections, though.

I read a lot of health-related books and magazines. Every day it seems there's something new to be found about nutrition, like:

- The health benefits of hot peppers.
- The wonderful omega-3 fatty acids.
- The power of antioxidants and phytochemicals in fruits and vegetables.
- Different sources of quality protein.
- The magic of fiber.

That list goes on and on. There's a cornucopia of health out there, waiting to be eaten. Just this morning while on the toilet I read a good article in *Runner's World* about many different edibles that reduce cholesterol, and while I was reading it, something clicked.

I have yet to read an article espousing the health benefits of Twinkies, Oreos, or Snickers. As a matter of fact, I'm going to go out on a limb here and state that I cannot remember reading a single article or study anywhere that indicates any real benefits from processed foods.

Whether you believe in God or you believe in evolution – or somewhere in between, perhaps – one fact is undeniable: our planet is loaded with extremely high-quality foods, all in their natural state. There are very few natural foods I can think of that are unhealthy, and even those have several benefits in reasonable quantities.

So much good nutrition waiting to improve our bodies, and we time and time again choose something that's prone to kill us in the long run. Why is that? Convenience, coupled with a lack of real concern for our health.

A common myth is that it is "too hard" to prepare quality meals regularly in today's hectic society. Baloney. Most fruits require little or no preparation. Wash it and eat it. Many vegetables are the same way, or if you'd prefer, there are all sorts of frozen vegetables just waiting to be steamed or microwaved. You can find all sorts of healthful whole-grain products at a "health-food" store or in the organic section of your supermarket.

For protein, eggs are incredibly simple to prepare. I like to break one into a bowl, stir it, and microwave it for one minute. How hard is that? Chicken is versatile and easy to cook, and you can prepare enough at once for several meals. Ditto for turkey, pork, and beef.

Sure, convenience foods are convenient. They didn't get that nickname because they're not. But a good number of them also make heart disease and obesity pretty convenient, too.

Is that what you want out of life?

November 27

Lots of people pack in food around holidays, simply because it's there. This year try something different. Think first. What's most important to you when the food's right in front of you? The taste? That taste is fleeting, and gone within minutes. Within hours, you'll defecate out what your body didn't digest or convert to fat.

Is it really worth it? The answer is not always "no." Sometimes the taste of the food is worth it – and that's fine. In like manner, the answer is not always "yes," either. It's not a problem until you find yourself eating everything, when nothing matters but shoving the food in your mouth.

The solution really is simple: be mindful. Think before you act, and realize that every action has a consequence. Choose wisely, and you won't have any problems at all.

November 30

Fat people have a love affair with numbers, to the point of obsession. Being concerned with numbers is fine; I guess my real beef is with *which* numbers we're so concerned.

The first number is the almighty scale number; all hail the scale! The scale tells your weight or, more accurately, it tells how much the earth's gravity is pulling your body toward the center of the earth. So what? What it *doesn't* tell is a thing about your health. Know what else it doesn't tell you? It doesn't tell you about your worth as a human. All too often we judge ourselves on what the scale says, and that's just plain self-defeating. The scale is not your judge or jury, it's simply a tool, and not a good tool at all for telling you how healthy you are.

People are also hooked on the number of pounds they've dropped. Sure, I've dropped 165 pounds, but that tells you nothing at all about whether I'm any healthier than I was eighteen months ago. Granted, since my number here is larger than the average person's I may not make the best example, but you get the point.

The third number people are obsessed with is a "goal weight." This one's not as bad as the first two, in my book, because we all need a target to aim for. My initial target was 175, then 185, and then 190 pounds, but as I grow healthier, I find that (a) I don't really know what the final number is going to be and (b) I don't really *care* what the final number is, because I'm concerned with different numbers. Numbers I think are more indicative of my overall health.

Numbers like my resting heart rate, which dropped from the low 90's to the low 50's over the last year and a half; like my blood cholesterol, which went from not too bad (157) to awesome (119) in that same time; like my triglycerides, which were in the 400s when I began, and were 76 the last time I had them checked; like my body fat, which is now in the teens, instead of being almost forty percent; like my blood sugar, which fell from 185 taking two pills a day to 66 with zero pills a day.

Do you see what I mean? Keep up with all the numbers you want to, but be mindful of what the numbers you're keeping really represent. Do they accurately show your health, or do they show something else?

December 2001

206 – 205 *pounds*

December 3

I've decided to answer the question I'm most often asked in my life, and I give it to you here as a sort of pocket reference.

Simple Secrets of Successful Weight Loss

The secret	The explanation
Eat to live; don't live to eat.	You control what you put into your mouth, no matter what you tell yourself about addictions or whatnot.
Don't starve.	As strange as it sounds, you have to eat to drop weight. Probably you should eat at the very minimum 10 calories per pound of your "goal" weight, and more per pound if you're active.
Move your butt.	Regularly. Be physical. Walk. Run. Play. Be creative, your body will thank you.

Move a little iron.	Lifting weights is one of the best things you can do for your body. Not only does it make you look better by firming and enlarging your muscles, it raises your resting metabolism round the clock.
Don't obsess.	Not over the scales, not about how much food you're eating, not about drinking 8 glasses of water a day. Everything in moderation. Eat plenty, drink plenty, move plenty.
Visualize.	See the person you want to be inside your head, and then live like that person. Watch yourself become that person.
Believe in yourself.	You're responsible for your every action, and anything you believe you can achieve, plain and simple.
Want it. Badly.	Anything you want, you can have. All you need is the desire to take it. The desire to transform can work wonders in the face of daily temptations – food sleep, laziness. How badly do you want it?
Stop making excuses and do it.	You know what I mean. Quit whining and shit or get off the pot.
Get busy living, or get busy dying.	Life's too short and precious to sit around not living it. I know, because I did that for ten years, and I miss those years. But I'm enjoying the hell out of the time I have left on this earth.

Eat whole.	Not the whole thing, but whole foods. Toss out the Slim-Fast and other such garbage, and eat whole foods. They're here for a reason. If you're going to have meal replacements, have a balanced one that doesn't get most of its calories/carbohydrates from sugar.
Eat natural.	I don't know a whole lot of fat people who eat 90+% of their foods from unprocessed sources. Lighten up on the junky and fast foods, and try some fruits, veggies, whole grains, nuts, and unprocessed meats. Your body loves them.
Can the pills.	You didn't need ephedra, or Xenical, or Meridia to get fat, did you? Here's my number one question for those of you taking pills to lose weight: What happens when you stop taking them?
Don't freak out.	A ten-pound gain in a day is NOT body fat; it is simply not possible. Stop worrying about it.
Really, don't freak out.	So you ate the Snickers, so what? The world didn't end, nor will it. We all make poor choices on occasion; the trick is to not do it that often.
Live as if.	Don't live like the fat person you are, that's what made you fat in the first place. Live like the person you want to be.

It's for the health, not the weight.	Dropping weight is a pleasant side effect of what the ultimate goal is: getting healthy. If you're just in it to drop a few pounds, go drink a Slim-Fast.
Stop trying.	Start doing.

December 6

Someone asked me today if people treat me differently now that I'm not fat. People treat me the same way as always, with one minor difference: they seem to look at me and smile at me a lot more. I'm not sure if they're really doing this, or if I'm simply paying more attention, but that's honestly the only real difference I see. That and the constant barrage of "how did you do it?" questions.

If I were a different person, say, one of those blamers we all know so well, I suppose I could claim that everyone was treating me differently because they'd discriminated against me for my fatness before, but we all know that's not true. Granted, people may notice you more in a physical sense because let's face it, whether it's right or wrong, in today's society fit and healthy is generally considered sexier than fat and dying.

The previous statements were regarding people who've known me both fat and fit. Strangers don't treat me any differently. Perhaps they don't stare as much, but then again, perhaps they weren't really staring before. Perhaps I only felt like they were staring because I was so freakishly fat.

As far as paying more attention, one thing I find about myself is that I'm looking at people more and smiling at them more, because my confidence level is much higher now, and I don't try to stay hidden in the back of the room. God knows I'd probably take off my clothes and pose for them if I thought I could get away with it. Interestingly, I keep expecting people – strangers – to stare at me these days, because I see the world differently now. To me (all ego aside here, even if I come across as sounding egotistical), I'm all hard-bodied and fit and good-looking, and I expect everyone to notice me and eyeball me appropriately. But they don't, and I think I've finally figured out why.

To them, I'm just another guy walking through the mall, tugging at his shirt nervously because he still thinks his man-boobs are jutting out. They don't know what I was; they only know what I am now, because to them I'm everyman.

To me, however, I'm something special.

December 8

One of the biggest reasons the vast majority of fat people never change is because they fear what the "sacrifices" are.

Listen closely. There are no sacrifices.

Why? Because it's not about the weight, it's about the health.

Think you cannot have Ben and Jerry's any more? You're wrong. You can have Ben and Jerry's, but you might not want to eat the whole container in one sitting. From a health perspective, you realize what some of the things – taken in excess – in Ben and Jerry's can do to your body, and you no longer want as much. It's not a matter of "can't have it," it's a matter of "don't want it."

Once you change your paradigm from a simple matter of weight to the more encompassing matter of total health, everything looks different. Food is not about what you can and cannot have; it is about what will best serve your body to make it healthier and stronger.

But, if you still want to look at it in terms of what you cannot have and what you can have, choose the positive. You can have a longer life, fewer medical problems, boundless energy and strength, and fun with life.

Or, you can choose to live in your shell, afraid of the "sacrifices," and have none of those.

Here are a few more things that make everything worth the effort:

- Sexual potency (being a male, I feel the need to list this first).
- The ability to climb a ladder.
- Fitting in almost anything designed for the average person. If there's something I don't fit in, it's because my shoulders are so broad, not because I'm fat.
- Not only being able to ride my daughter's scooter, but being able to ride said scooter without worrying about breaking it.
- Only being able to get out of breath by making a concerted effort.

- Not straining to replace the 5-gallon water bottle at work.
- Feeling more refreshed on less sleep.
- Not getting sick every few months.
- Confidence.
- Appreciative looks from women.
- Being proud of my body, rather than ashamed.
- Not losing my mind if I have to remove my shirt in front of someone.
- Being able to run again.
- Not worrying about my weight.
- No diabetes.
- Low cholesterol.
- A resting heart rate in the low 50s.
- Knees that work properly again (loud grinding from years of abuse because of my fatness notwithstanding).
- Knowing that I can help in an emergency, not bound or slowed by being fat.
- Not being the biggest person in the room, or even close.
- Having anyone – except the smallest child – be able to completely wrap their arms around me when they hug me.
- Not having people feel sorry for me because I'm fat.
- Not having well-meaning friends try to advise me on "weight loss."
- Having less healthy friends now coming to me for advice on getting healthy.
- Running up the stairs with a 20-pound bag of cat food in one hand and a 20-pound bucket of cat litter in the other, and still not breathing hard.
- Mobility.
- Being able to reach every part of my body.
- Being able to see every part of the front of my body.
- Being able to cut my own toenails.
- Not getting constipated because of all the crappy food I ate.
- Never having to stop and rest.
- Not feeling like people are staring at me

- Not being embarrassed to go in public places.
- Wearing t-shirts.
- Shopping anywhere I please for clothes.
- Having clothes cost less, because they're not abnormally sized.
- Watching old friends do double takes when they see me – or having them not recognize me at all.
- Bike riding.
- Having my daughter tell me that when she took a "muscle-flexing" picture of me to school for art class, the whole class oohed and ahhed when she showed it as her example.
- No more yeast infections.
- No odors from places where fat rolls sweated.
- Feeling my ribs, hips, and other various bones.
- Seeing my face look human again.
- Realizing that I can accomplish anything I choose, if only I believe in myself.

Are you convinced yet that it's worth the "sacrifice"?

December 13

We'll be right back after these messages…

And now, a few words from our sponsors…

Don't touch that dial! Our show will return shortly…

We've all heard these words, and we all know what they mean. Commercials. Thirty-second television spots designed to make us buy a particular product, or call a particular lawyer, or eat at a particular restaurant.

They can make us laugh, and they can make us cry. The one thing the advertisers hope they can do is convince us to select what they're selling.

Last night, Robyn and I spent our evening in front of the television, and we saw plenty of commercials. In betwixt the car ads and the clothes ads, there were food ads. Lots of food ads, and something jumped out at me all of the sudden. Perhaps I'm slow, being from Alabama and all, and maybe all of you have known it for years, but it just became obvious to me last night.

Food advertised on television is not even remotely good for you.

Of course I have examples – the commercials I remember from just last night. Most restaurants post nutritional information, and if I couldn't find what I wanted, I didn't hesitate to call their customer service numbers in my quest to find information.

First up is Arby's. Those guys are having a special right now, four Beef-n-Cheddar sandwiches for a reduced price. What they don't tell you is that each sandwich loads you up with four hundred eighty calories. Assuming you only have one, and throw in a regular order of curly fries for another 400 calories, you can grab a quick lunch at Arby's for about 900 calories, if you drink water or Diet Coke.

Oh yeah, 400 of the calories are from fat. Fat is not bad, but I'm betting most of this fat *is not* omega-3 or mono- and poly-unsaturated fats, which your body loves.

Next up was Domino's, who pointed out that I should give my kids the taste they love, and purchase for them a bacon cheeseburger pizza. If you want one, a single slice of a 12-inch hand-tossed one is two hundred eighty calories. But really, who eats one piece? We all eat more like three or four pieces at a time.

Hardees pitched their six-dollar burger, which weighs in at nine hundred forty nine calories. Pick up a regular fries and regular Coke to round out your meal with an additional five hundred forty five calories.

Do you see a pattern yet?

The last advertiser I recall was Pizza Hut, selling their new Ultimate Meat Lover's Pizza, a mix of – get ready, I had to call customer service for this – pepperoni, Italian sausage, ham, pork, bacon, and beef, topped off with mozzarella, Romano, Monterey jack, Parmesan, provolone, and cheddar cheeses.

Holy cow.

This baby – in the hand-tossed version – has three hundred thirty calories in a single slice, and seven grams of the artery-killer, saturated fat. Again, like Domino's: who eats one slice?

If there's one thing that really stands out, it's this: I cannot find one single redeeming thing (nutritionally speaking) about any of the foods that were pushed on me last night. It wouldn't be a problem if people had these foods occasionally, but let's face it, most Americans eat out at least once a day, and most of them choose a place like one mentioned above to eat.

Sure I sound anal, but you've come to expect that of me.

Wake up, America, and smell what's getting shoveled in front of you. Stop being a sheep to the advertisers. They want you to think that your kids will play more if they eat a bacon cheeseburger pizza from Domino's, or that you can get a "restaurant experience without the restaurant" from Hardees. They want you to think that your life will be improved if you eat their food, and you believe them, and buy it.

Don't get me wrong, I've been there. I remember ordering – and eating entire – meat lover's pizzas from Pizza Hut. I remember buying Arby's 5 for $5 special (I didn't like beef-n-cheddar; I liked regulars) and eating all five in one sitting. So don't think I'm sitting on a high horse here, looking down. I've been there.

It comes down to a simple question: what do you want out of life, and what are you willing to do to get it? The choices are yours.

December 15

If you look at one of my typical days now, as compared to one of my typical days when I was fat, there might not be a lot of obvious differences. I eat more often now, five or six times a day. I drink more water and less carbonated drinks now than I did.

I sleep less now, and I feel more rested and refreshed since I don't toss and turn all night. I roll out of bed much faster, and though I enjoy a good afternoon snooze on the weekend, I no longer require daily naps.

Obviously, another difference is that I work out in the mornings now instead of lying in bed, but what I've listed are the only real daily differences visible to the naked eye. There's another huge difference between the old Fred and the new Fred, one that you cannot see just by looking at a typical day. You see it when you look at the overall picture of the way my life is now as opposed to the way it was.

That difference is *potential.* I have no limits now, where before I was constantly limited by my size, my fitness, and my shame.

If I wanted to throw the Frisbee or football in the field behind my office, I couldn't. Now I can. If I wanted to take my daughter to the park and play on the playground, I couldn't. Now I can. If wanted to get undressed in front of a masseuse, I couldn't. Now I can. My potential now versus my potential then is the single biggest difference in my life because that potential is what changes "I cannot" into "I can."

And that kicks butt.

December 16

Here is a great truth I've discovered over the last 18 months: a lot of fat people are in denial. Not in denial about being fat, they realize that part, but in denial over how easy it is to remedy the problem. I have a theory about the mental processes behind this, which I'd like to share. This is what I think is happening inside the mind of a typical fat person:

"If it's easy to get rid of this extra weight/fat, I'd have done it by now. I've tried plenty of diets, and none of them worked for me, or if they did, I got re-fatted as soon as I stopped following them. Therefore, since I'm still fat (or fat again), it must be hard to make myself unfat."

Taking the logic a step further, "Because it's so hard to get rid of all this fat/weight, the only thing that must work is something radical, like a pill or surgery or starvation."

I experience a lot of backlash over what I've done because I have the unmitigated gall to have done it in a most healthy manner, rather quickly, while preaching all along how easy it is (was) to do it. I've been accused of lying (this is the most popular accusation, for the record), of starving myself, of taking "metabolism boosters," and of editing pictures of myself. I've been asked if I've had gastric bypass surgery, if I have cancer, if I have AIDS, and if I'm on prescription medications or liquid diets.

No one wants to believe the simple answer – that I stopped eating so much garbage and got my butt in motion – because of the whole "if it's that simple, I wouldn't be fat" mentality. On occasion that frustrates me, because I feel like I've found the answer to one of life's big issues, and all I want to do is share it with people.

December 17

Somewhere over the last couple of months, I became able to do something I've never done in my entire life: pull-ups. Not one, not two, but three at a time. My door gym caught my eye last night and I thought, *I haven't tried a pull-up in a while, maybe I could do one now.* So I tried, and found that I could. I called the wife and daughter up to see, and demonstrated for them. I wasn't wearing a shirt, and Danielle complained that when I did a pull-up, my back got "all gross and lumpy." I'll take that as a compliment.

December 18

If you're on a limited budget and don't think it's possible to eat both cheap and healthy, consider:

- Water-packed tuna is extremely healthy, and is less than a dollar a can.
- Dried beans are just over fifty cents a pound.
- Brown rice is a dollar for two pounds, and makes a complete protein source when mixed with beans.
- Eggs are ninety cents a dozen – scramble 1 whole and 5 or 6 whites, and you've got a nice protein mix.
- Pasta is cheap, and a reasonably decent complex carbohydrate.
- Frozen vegetables are a dollar or less a bag, usually.
- In the summer months roadside produce is very inexpensive.
- Whole chickens and chicken parts are pretty cheap.
- Ground beef is inexpensive. Just rinse it after you cook it, to wash away some of the unhealthier fats.

For dinner tonight our main course was black beans and rice with a couple of chicken breasts thrown in for additional protein. The cost? About $2.50 to feed the three of us, and I have three lunches to take to work out of that single pot.

Never think you don't have enough money to buy healthy foods.

Speaking from experience, I can remember how much the comments from my friends and family hurt when they were trying to be helpful, back in the days when I was super fat. I'm betting most of you know what I'm talking about, because you've had those same comments made to you.

"You could really be good looking if you lost a little weight." Ironically, I find that that one turned out to be true.

"You won't ever find a girlfriend if you keep eating like that."

"You're eating yourself into an early grave."

"I'm afraid you're going to die."

The list goes on. Every single one came from a well-meaning person, and every single one didn't work. As painful as it may be, only you can be responsible for changing yourself.

That said, you can always lead by example and hope that something triggers a change in the person, but here's something else you might not want to hear: the person in question might be perfectly happy with himself/herself. Just because you think they should lose weight, get fit, whatever, doesn't mean that they think so.

December 19

Regularly people on "low-carbohydrate diets" ask me how I can eat so many carbohydrates and still get rid of fat. I can do it for one simple reason: I consume less energy than I expend.

Carbohydrates can make you fat, that's a true statement. So can protein, and so can fat. It's entirely possible, if you're really dedicated, to get fat eating nothing but salad. No single food is the culprit. Too much food is, plain and simple.

Don't be swept up by the fad diet of the week. There's a reason they're called "fad" diets.

The driving force (generally) behind the carbohydrates I choose to eat boils down to a single question: will it help my body or hurt my body? I aim for eating foods that will help me most of the time, and tend to minimize the hurtful foods. I eat things I enjoy, like whole grains, fruits, and lots of vegetables for carbohydrates.

Mostly I strive to eat unprocessed foods. As for telling if something's processed, there are a couple of general rules that help. First, if it comes in a wrapper, it's been processed. Not necessarily a lot, but some. The real question to ask is this: how close is the food to its natural state? The closer it is to being natural, the better it probably is for you.

Take wheat for example. In the natural state, you have whole or cracked grain. Generally, by the time I get it, it's been ground (more processing) and mixed into whole wheat bread. After that stage, all the fiber and vitamins have been processed out and it has been bleached to make soft (read: nutritionally void) white flour. The worst part is that bakers then have to add back the vitamins they stripped out in a process they call "enriching" the flour.

Point to remember: The closer it is to its natural state, the better it probably is for you.

December 20

Today, a co-worker brought in candy. Lots of it: mini Reese's cups, mini Almond joys, Hershey's miniatures, and mini $100,000 bars. He put them in a big jar in his office, and invited everyone to partake.

So I partook. Twice. Handfuls.

A little background, though. Today is a no-exercise day, so I didn't have my post-workout shake. Things were hectic at work, and I ended up not eating breakfast until about eleven. Since it was the first I'd had to eat, I was pretty hungry.

Not that I'm making an excuse, because excuses are bullshit.

I ate a bunch of candy right after breakfast because I was still hungry. So much candy, in fact, that I wasn't hungry at lunchtime. I didn't get hungry until about 4:30, actually.

Now there's proof positive I don't eat like an anal retentive all the time.

Pay attention, though, because there's a lesson here. I won't look back, and I won't regret or feel bad for what I did. The world's not ending because I ate candy, and I'm no less healthy for having done it. Don't kill yourself over one small bad choice, because one bad choice cannot hurt you. Just don't create a pattern. You don't get fat from an incident, you get fat when you consistently have these incidents.

December 22

Something horrible happened to me this morning on my walk-jog. Something traumatic, and I don't know if I'll ever be the same again.

It happened during a walking period. I was making my circuit around the local middle school while it was still dark, as is my habit, and I was deep into the audio book I'm currently listening to. I was moving at a goodly clip, breathing strongly and enjoying the story playing out in my ears.

My foot rolled on and kicked something in the middle of my stride. Hard.

I looked down to see what I'd kicked and saw, to my horror, the body of a cute little mouse flipping and flopping across the parking lot, its tail flailing loosely. It stopped and didn't move. I felt horrible. I felt wicked. I felt *evil.*

I stepped over to the mouse's limp body and knelt, hoping beyond hope it might be okay. It lay still as I moved closer, without even a twitch from its tail. I didn't want to touch it – diseases and all that – but it was damn hard to see because it was so dark. I lowered my face a little closer and found that I'd been mistaken.

It wasn't a mouse at all; it was a tampon.

A *soiled* tampon.

Ugh.

December 23

As of yesterday, I've officially kept 100 pounds of fat off my body for one year.

Where I work, I get paid every two weeks. Out of every check, I have a percentage of money withheld and split among several mutual funds, so that I'll have plenty of money available when I retire. I daresay a good number of people do the exact same thing. After all, who wants to have to work until they die because they failed to set aside money when they were able?

We invest money for our retirement, but we don't invest time in taking care of ourselves: feeding our body proper nutrition and working it regularly. Instead, we grab a fast food meal on the go, because we "don't have time" to prepare healthful foods. We plan to go to the gym to work out, but again we suddenly find that we don't have time.

Know something? If you don't take the time today to prepare for your future health, you're going to find you might not have a future. I don't mean to sound melodramatic there, but it's a fact: unhealthy people die young. Live for the moment, but prepare for the future. You're worth the investment in yourself.

December 24

Do you think, had you not ever watched that emergency room documentary, that today you would still be the old Fred, or do you think you would have begun your transformation to the new Fred by now anyway?

Someone asked me one of those "what if" questions today, so let me state up front that everything pertaining to this particular question is pure conjecture.

I believe that the documentary in question was a catalyst, rather than a complete causative. Remember, the day I saw the show on TV, we'd just returned from our first vacation in a while, from Gatlinburg, Tennessee. On that trip I'd had a very rude awakening, because there were several things pushed to the front of my thinking that I'd been successfully not thinking about for many years. Things like:

I could only walk about a block at a time before I had to stop and sit for a while, due to the pain in my left ankle.

I couldn't fit on most of the rides there, and the ones I did fit on – a virtual roller and a motion theater ride – bruised me something awful because I was too big for them.

I couldn't keep up with my daughter.

I had to stop several times on the 4.5-hour drive home to pee, because of my blood sugar.

Robyn and I did more sitting around than anything; it was like we weren't even on vacation.

While I wasn't thinking, *hey, I need to get my fat ass into shape or I'm going to die*, or anything like that, there were several mitigating factors leading up to the incident with the show. In essence, I was primed and ready, and the show was the final thing that started the fire in my head.

I guess what I'm saying is that I was ready, and if I hadn't seen the show, something else would've happened. I'm just thankful it wasn't a heart attack.

❦

I'm hearing a lot of the same things from my overweight friends these days, dreams and promises waiting to be smashed on the reality of life. This is what they sound like:

I'm going to lose weight as soon as the holidays are over.

I've been off track over the holidays, but I'll get right back on after Christmas.

I'm miserable with the way I've been eating since Thanksgiving. I cannot wait for January so I can get back into groove.

I know what these are, because I said the very same things for many years. I know all about breaking promises to myself.

Let me ask a question: if you're not willing to change yourself right now, what makes you think you'll be willing to change yourself next week?

It's not meant to be a rude question, but it's the truth. I'm not advocating doing something Draconian for Christmas, like eating a piece of lettuce while everyone else feasts on ham, cakes, casseroles, and whatnot. Just keep in mind that this season is about family and friends, and for many people it's also a celebration of their faith.

It's not about the food.

Food is a part of it, yes, because the human social condition generally requires food to be present at any gathering. Just remember that food's not the main part of it. In this season of giving, give something to yourself: a longer, more healthful life.

December 27

I've discovered some of the emotional baggage that comes with making a significant body transformation. I use the word "emotional" loosely, because I cannot think of a better one. What I've found is this:

On days when I choose to eat extra food, or food that's not so healthy, and on days where I don't work out at all (like today, actually), I have spastic moments of concern where I feel like I'm going to magically transform back into the pre-May-2000 Fred. Logically – and I'm generally a very logical person – I realize that this is impossible; I know in my head that even if I pigged out every day on the worst junk food I could find, and didn't work out for an entire week, that I might add back five pounds of fat. More realistically, I'm betting I'd only add back a couple.

That's what I know in my head. In my heart, however, I'm concerned that it's all over, that I'm going to catch sight of myself in the mirror and find that I'm suddenly a big blob again, that one day of inactivity will be the end of me.

Ah, neurosis.

Let me stress something here: this is not as bad as it might sound. Please don't think I turn into a quivery pile of Jell-o, because I don't. It's more a random thought than any sort of real concern, so don't be thinking I'm losing my mind or anything.

At least, losing the mind I have left.

December 30

I'm pleased to announce that I ran my entire new cardio route today – two and a half miles – without stopping to walk once. Not that I'm planning to make that regular or anything, but it's still a first. I'm constantly amazed at how much my body can adapt and recover on my days off. And speaking of my days off...

❧

Robyn and I were talking and laughing this morning about the exercise we used to do. When we started exercising, we started together, in early June of 2000. Somewhere around the 6th or 7th, if memory serves.

Note: we were laughing at ourselves, because we've come so far, not to poke fun at the amount of exercise anyone does. We all have starting points – some of you may start out in better shape than I did (hell, some of you probably started out in better shape than I'm in *now*), some of you may start out in worse shape. The shape you're in doesn't matter, as long as you start. You'll improve over time, guaranteed, and then you can look back and laugh because you've come so far.

My very first exercise was running in place on the slope between the shallow end and the deep end in our pool for ten minutes, after which I was panting like a racehorse. Robyn did basically the same thing next to me. After a few weeks, I'd worked up to 20 or so minutes on the stationary bike. In my very first exercise log entry, written for June 25, 2000, this is what I said:

For exercise today, I rode my stationary bike for 21:06. I rode 5.0 miles, and if the meter on the bike is to be believed, I burned 150 calories. My butt was asleep when I finished.

See what I mean about laughing? I gradually moved over to walking with videos, and worked my way up to 3 or 4 miles a day indoors with those. At the end of August 2000, I decided to lift weights. For two days, then I quit – because I was afraid it would slow my pound-dropping progress. Here's what I said in my journal at the time:

It would appear that the vast majority of the people I know think I should continue lifting weights, for a variety of reasons. Most prevalent is that weight training will raise my metabolism, and help me to shed weight faster. The second most popular idea is that I'm currently shedding muscle mass because I'm not weight training, and that if I do begin the training, I'll stop dropping muscle.

Forgive me if I disagree, but I have a goal to keep.

See? I made mistakes along the way. No one is perfect, and don't let anyone ever tell you that you *should* be.

At the beginning of September 2000, I walked outside for the first time. I humped it for a whole hour, because I thought I was in good shape, and I made it 3.3 miles in that hour. The next day, I had plenty to say:

I learned a great truth this morning when I got out of bed. I realized that walking for real and walking with tapes are FAR from being the same. I haven't hurt so much since Bill Clinton won the presidency in 1992.

It wouldn't be so bad if it were only my legs (every single muscle in them, apparently), but my back hurts too, all the way up to my shoulder blades. My lower back hurts the most; it actually aches even when I'm not doing anything, but really flares up nicely when I get up and walk around.

In January 2001, I decided to start lifting weights again, because I felt that with having dropped over a hundred pounds, I was no longer "too fat" to lift. My first chest workout involved five sets of chest presses and one set of flyes. In that first workout, I moved 2600 pounds of weight on my home gym with my chest.

Today I moved 9250 pounds of free weight with my chest, then followed up with biceps work and ran for two and a half miles.

Your body longs to be worked. You might not believe it now, if you haven't worked it in a while, but it does. And when you work it, it will respond by transforming in front of your very eyes – if you're in the poor shape I once was, you'll see changes almost every single day.

Give your body what it wants, and taste the freedom of fitness.

December 31

I write a lot about transforming, because I believe a transformation is necessary if you want to make a permanent lifelong change. At the end of Webster's definition of the word "transform" is the following: "*Transform implies a major change in form, nature, or function.*"

This is the time of year when people are looking back over the last year of broken health promises, and making new promises to "lose weight" or "get in shape" in 2002. Often, these people will succumb to the garbage they see on the television or hear on the radio, in hopes that they might find something – some small bit of magic – that will transform them into the person they long to be.

That's how companies stay in business selling abdominal shockers that promise to give you a six-pack. That's what keeps the Hollywood Diet – *lose 10 pounds in 48 hours!* – going. That's why people buy vibrating belts that can "take inches" off their midsections, or pills that make you "lose weight while you sleep."

Garbage, all of it. Let's talk about *real* transformation.

A real transformation begins on the inside, not in a bottle or a package. The magic is sitting inside you, waiting to be let out. The transformation is a learning process, one that comes from realizing you control your destiny and that you can accomplish whatever you decide you're going to accomplish. You cannot get that from a toll-free number.

The transformation begins simply, with nothing more than a decision to raise your standards and no longer accept the life you've been living. Follow the decision with actions – eat natural, eat plenty, and move plenty – and watch your body change as your whole perspective on life changes.

I've changed pretty dramatically since I began, on both the outside and the inside. The external changes are obvious, so I won't go into them.

I changed from being someone who went out of his way to avoid physical activity to being someone who not only looks forward to physical activity, but who now goes out of his way to do things. I went from being someone who thought he was "too fat" to lift weights to someone who absolutely loves weightlifting. I now dislike foods I once loved, and love foods I once disliked. In short, I'm a whole new man: new looks, new attitudes, new emotions, and new priorities for my life.

Something you buy from an infomercial is not going to transform you, because it doesn't teach you anything. You don't learn from them, unless it's learning that buying them is a mistake. Trust me, I've bought enough of them to know.

Transformation does not depend on what the scales tell you. Your mystical "goal weight" – which I once had, too – is nothing more than an ideal. I weigh over 200 pounds right now, yet am considerably smaller than I was in high school, when I weighed 196. I'm also in much better shape, and have a lot more muscle mass. I've harped on it plenty, because it's a very important concept: don't let the scales determine your self worth.

Treat yourself better. Toss the fads, forget the scales, and make a commitment to yourself. Living healthy is not nearly as hard as you've programmed yourself to think and you'll get back so much more than you put in that I don't think I could begin to list all the benefits – though I've tried in several entries. You're worth the commitment to, because we're all worth the commitment to live a long and healthy life.

January 2002

205 – 204 *pounds*

January 5

I have a love/hate relationship with the day of the week when I don't work out. I love the day because my body uses the time to repair itself, and I'll ultimately be stronger tomorrow, when I pound my chest and biceps. That is a wonderful thing.

I hate the day because I feel like I'm making no progress when I just sit around on my ass. Yes, I know it's illogical, but I'm not talking logic right now. I don't quite think I'm talking emotion, either, I think maybe it's more like the soft, silent voice of irrationality.

He's an insidious bastard, irrationality. He tells you things you know aren't true, and yet you want to believe him. For example, one of the biggest things he whispers to me is that if I'm not lifting, I'm not getting more muscle mass. This is a lie, because you don't build muscle when you're lifting weights, you tear it down. Your muscles actually get bigger while you're resting, because your body is repairing them. Hence the recommendations to always give a muscle group at least 24 hours between workouts.

So I sit here on my non-lifting days, knowing logically that those are the best days for making me more buff since my body is using that downtime to rebuild, but that little bastard whispers in my head, *C'mon, Fred, it won't hurt to do a few pull-ups, or maybe some pushups. You can't just sit here all day, that's what made you so fat in the first place, remember?*

My guess is that I'm not alone in hearing the voice of irrationality. Have no fear if you hear that little voice in your head on your non-workout days: you're not alone.

Just ignore the little bastard. You need to rest.

❧

Okay, here's a tidbit for the water-obsessed among us. I say that tongue-in-cheek because it is my considered opinion that no one is as obsessive about water as a fat person. One would think, from watching in chats, reading message boards, and eavesdropping on conversations that water was the second coming.

It's not.

It's important, yes, and I believe we should drink plenty of it. I just don't think we need to be counting out our 8 glasses and all that. Just drink it.

People ask me regularly how much water I drink. The simple answer is this: I don't know, because I don't count it. Life is too short for that. However, this is what I can tell you: by 8 am most days, I've already consumed more than the recommended 8 glasses. Therefore, if we extrapolate, I'd guess probably close to a gallon of water a day. Add to that a whole pot of coffee, part of a sugar-free root beer with lunch, and several 32-oz glasses of tea and/or lemonade at night, and I'm pretty well hydrated.

And no, I don't believe the baloney about caffeinated drinks dehydrating you; there are no studies that conclusively show that. From what I've read, most people build up a tolerance to caffeine pretty quickly and the effects become negligible. However, don't start drinking caffeinated drinks exclusively. For drinking, nothing's as good for you as pure water.

January 6

My "rules" for myself haven't really changed from the beginning. The only hard and fast rules I made were that I would put myself – my health – first, and that I would be true to myself. That hasn't changed at all. Some of the things I do have changed, and mistakes have been made along the way.

A couple that come to mind: my resistance to weight lifting until I "wasn't so fat" and my obsession with the numbers on the scale, both of which I've written about recently so I won't go over those again. I will say this: I understand people's obsession with the scale, I just wish I could find a good way to get across how unimportant it really is in the grand scheme of things.

Both realizations caused me to modify what I was doing, because they changed my perception of the man I wanted to be. Originally, I had this idea that I wanted to be a fit and healthy 190-pound man. Not a bad goal, but perhaps not reasonable, because I didn't realize at the beginning just how much I was going to enjoy weight training. Now, I don't know if I'll get below 200, and you know what?

I don't care.

See, at the beginning, I said it was all about the health, but in retrospect I think a good bit of it was really about the weight. I attached an arbitrary weight to the man I wanted to be, and I focused on that. At some point (I cannot pinpoint it, unfortunately), health really did become the focus, and as a result, I stopped eating as much junky food as I did at the beginning and started eating unprocessed foods almost exclusively. Getting information about what companies put into their food is a big eye opener.

Also along the way I realized that the man I wanted to be probably weighed more than 190, because he was (is) a well-muscled man. That realization is the source of my recent "ditch the scales" soapbox, because as I've said, the scale cannot accurately determine your health, unless you are still seriously fat.

January 9

I joined a Weight Watchers chat today, and I stayed there for about an hour just watching the conversation.

Holy cow.

Weight Watchers, in its intended form, can be a helpful tool for people who need to drop excess fat. In essence, you get a certain number of "points" you can ingest each day (a number that's low, in the not-so-humble opinion of your author, particularly for someone working on becoming fit at the same time) which pretty much limits the number of calories you can have. Nice and simple.

Almost. Like any tool, the Weight Watchers point system can be abused. For the entire chat, the conversation centered around two things: points and eating.

The points talk all centered around how many points a particular food had. Bacon, pizza, and ham were the top three subjects discussed, and how much of each one could have for how many points. People discussed how you could get the maximum pizza for the fewest points, or which brands of bacon had the least points. Much discussion was had over no-point foods, yet in the entire hour I was there, there wasn't a single mention of a vegetable, a whole grain, a fruit, or even an unprocessed meat.

Oatmeal was mentioned a few times, as a breakfast food, but only in the context of being the kind of oatmeal you get out of a packet. Oh, and the discussions about how you could add cocoa and powdered peanut butter to it, because they're fat free.

What the hell is powdered peanut butter?

The eating talk was constant. What everyone had for breakfast, what everyone was having for lunch, and what everyone was having for dinner. The eating talk was coupled with the points talk, of course, and meals were all defined not by their contents or nutritional value, but by their points. Great deals of time were expended confessing "eating sins," like pigging out at Pizza Hut last night until spontaneous vomiting occurred.

Occasionally, physical activity was mentioned, usually walking or Richard Simmons videos (not that there is anything wrong with those, but we know cardio alone doesn't cut it). In one of the instances where I spoke in the chat, I asked if anyone did resistance training. Out of the entire room, one person (myself excluded) did, "sometimes." Mostly, though, they talked about eating and points.

Oh, man, and numbers. I forgot all about the numbers. People made the number of pounds they'd dropped part of their name, and went on and on about how weigh-in was tomorrow, or the next day, and oh how they'd been so "bad" and how their "fingers were crossed" that they wouldn't show a gain.

Listen closely.

Life is about so much more than this. Transforming yourself from fat and dying to fit and living is not about how much food you can sneak in, or about how little you can be active, or about some number on a scale. That's not transforming, that's imprisoning. Freedom is so much better. Having the mentality that you cannot have anything "good" or that you have to "suffer" through exercising is why so many fat people stay fat. They don't liberate themselves; they chain themselves down with some hellacious rules and ideas.

Here's a fact: if you're following the points system, you *cannot* have a lot of pizza, because pizza's mostly nutritionally void. Spending your time trying to figure out the maximum amount of garbage you can ingest for the least calories is a losing process, because you're still eating garbage. Consider: for considerably less calories than 2 pieces of pepperoni hand-tossed pizza, you can have a whole wheat pita with tomato sauce, diced chicken, a pile of fresh veggies, and cheese. Add to it a big salad and a piece of fruit, and you've got a pretty decent meal, all for fewer calories and a whole lot more nutrition.

This is one of the reasons I don't have to bother with counting calories or points or anything – I eat mostly natural foods, and natural foods are, well, naturally more healthful and less calorically dense. I'm not being smug here, and I'm not bragging. I simply feel very strongly about natural foods. I've eaten plenty of garbage, and I've seen firsthand what it can do to a perfectly good body. Free yourself from the prison of trying to squeeze in as much trash with the least calories, and come find out what health and vitality are all about.

January 11

We're many days into the year now, and the advertising onslaught has begun. You know what I'm talking about – the fat DJ's on the radio who are going to use metabolism boosters, again. The ads for products claiming to burn fat while you sleep. And lest I forget, there are now devices to deliver electric shocks to your abdomen to give you a six-pack.

You're being hit from every side right now by people who want your money.

Don't believe the hype – if something sounds too good to be true, it usually is. You know how to take charge of your life and transform yourself into the person you want to be, all you have to do is make the commitment to yourself and believe in yourself enough to keep your commitment.

January 18

In Japanese, the word *nintai* is written with two characters. The first character, *nin*, means "to bear silently," and the second character, *tai*, means "to endure with great patience." The English translation of *nintai* is "perseverance." It means, simply, to not give up. The only impossible things are the things you make impossible.

Every major religion teaches perseverance. In Christianity, Paul exhorts the Hebrews to "persevere so that when you have done the will of God, you will receive what he has promised." (Hebrews 10:36, NIV) The Koran calls Muslims to "seek Allah's help with patient perseverance" (S2 V45), and Buddha teaches his followers to "persevere in thy quest and thou shalt find what thou seekest." (The Renunciation)

Abraham Lincoln was born into poverty in a log cabin. Over the years, he lost eight elections, suffered a nervous breakdown, and failed in business not once but twice. Yet we remember none of this, save the log cabin. Why? Because Lincoln persevered. He endured, and he didn't give up, and he's considered one of the greatest presidents America has ever had.

Thomas Edison invented numerous items we still use: the phonograph, the mimeograph, and the movie projector. He patented over 1000 inventions in his life all in all, and he's known as the "Wizard of Menlo Park." Most people don't remember those facts, though. They remember that Edison invented the light bulb, which we have because Edison persevered. He tried 10,000 different ways to make the incandescent bulb work before he was able to. When asked why he kept trying after so many failures, he said (paraphrased), "I haven't failed 10,000 times, I have found 10,000 ways that don't work."

To persevere is to not give up. No matter how difficult something is, no matter how long it takes, and no matter who tells you it is impossible.

Lance Armstrong won the Tour de France after nearly dying from cancer. Harlan Sanders had almost 5000 people reject his recipe for fried chicken. Daniel "Rudy" Ruettiger fought nearly impossible odds to attend Notre Dame and play football, and in his single play in his only game, he sacked the opposing team's quarterback and was carried off the field on his teammates' shoulders.

Physical transformation takes time, and it takes patience. Enduring patience. Perseverance. You didn't get out of shape and unhealthy overnight, and you won't get fit and healthy overnight – despite what the infomercials tell you.

To persevere is to not give up. No matter how difficult your transformation is, no matter how long it takes, and no matter who tells you it is impossible.

January 23

It is official, as of my trip to JC Penney yesterday. Excepting my loose and floppy t-shirts I wear around the house, my wardrobe is X-free, size-wise. No more XL shirts, no more XL sweats or pants. I bought five new pastel shirts: lavender, green, yellow, blue, and pink. All sized "L."

It looks like the lawsuits may be coming soon. Sue McDonald's because you got fat eating their Big Macs. Give me a break. Let's sue Jack Daniels because some people drink too much of their whiskey. And while we're at it, let's sue Smith and Wesson because people get shot with their guns. Oh wait, we already did that.

Can I sue Pacific Fitness because I pulled a muscle in my back using equipment they made? Never mind the fact that I leaned forward and lifted my butt off the seat when I was lowering the weight, it wasn't my fault.

Welcome to America, the land of the victim.

Let me open the box of truth and share something with you: you, me, us, we are 100% responsible for what we put into our mouths at any given time. Period.

Yes, the fast food industry bombards us constantly, but that doesn't mean we have to run after them like lemmings to the sea. Take charge of your life, take responsibility for your actions, and either stop buying the crap or stop complaining about being fat.

The only reason McDonald's spent $500,000,000 on the "We love to see you smile" campaign is *because it works*. It works because we don't care enough about our bodies to give them proper nutrition. "Convenience" wins out over "healthy" all the time in this country, and our bellies show it.

All it takes to change the pattern is for you to engage your brain before you engage your mouth. I'm not saying, "don't ever eat a Big Mac again," I'm merely suggesting that eating them every day for lunch can have a definite adverse effect on your girth and health. It's all about the choices you make, and the responsibility you take for yourself.

Did you know that after age 25, a person who doesn't lift weights can lose up to one-half pound of muscle each year? Have you pumped your iron today?

January 25

Most of us have, sitting in our garages or driveways, at least one automobile. It might be an old car; it might be a new car. It could be a luxury car; it could be an economy car. Perhaps it's a large car; perhaps it's a small car. It is *your* car, and my guess is that you take pretty good care of it. You wash it and wax it, keep it fairly clean, and take it in for regular maintenance at a service station.

You also have a body. There are many similarities between our bodies and our automobiles, and I'm thinking of a few of them today.

Our bodies need fuel just like our cars do. We have to refuel both on a regular basis, and the way each "runs" is entirely dependent upon the sort of fuel we put in to it. For example, if I take my Jeep to Bubba's Cheep Gas and fill up, my fuel lines get gummed up, the engine knocks, and the Jeep drives erratically until I fuel up with better gas. When I fill the Jeep with Amoco Premium, it surges with acceleration and moves like greased lightning.

If I fill my body with junk food as I once did, it moves slowly. The fuel lines get gummed up, my heart knocks, and I feel like crap until I use better fuel. When I load up with fresh fruits, whole grains, lean meats, and vegetables, my body surges with power: I can run farther, lift more, and work harder. The quality of your fuel determines the quality of your body.

Like my Jeep, certain fuels tend to make my body backfire, too.

Oil – grease – is the lubricant for your automobile. It keeps the moving pieces moving smoothly, and prevents breakdowns from friction. Without proper lubrication, your car dries up and breaks down, often times permanently. Our bodies need a lubricant too, to run properly. It's water. Without water we break down permanently. Water keeps our joints functioning properly, keeps our digestive tract moving, filters poisons out of us, and is a part of every system in our bodies. There's no perfect substitute for pure water.

The heart of your car is the engine. When the engine stops, the car stops. Preventative maintenance in the form of oil changes, good gas, tune-ups, and so on ensure that your car's engine runs well for years. Your body's heart will run well for many years, too, with proper preventative maintenance: regular aerobic activity, good fuel, and periodic checkups from your family body mechanic.

In your automobile's engine, the pistons are responsible for transmitting the engine's combustion force to the crankshaft, and thus driving movement. The pistons take an immense amount of abuse, because they have to stop and start quickly, and deliver tremendous force. For an engine to run properly, all the pistons must move in perfect harmony. Our bodies have muscles to perform the same task. Muscular contractions cause all the movement in our bodies, and for our bodies to move lithely and quickly, muscular training is necessary.

The list of analogies goes on: wheels and legs, radiators and sweating, electrical system and nervous system are just a few that come to mind.

There is one striking difference between our bodies and our cars, however. Our bodies can repair the damage we inflict on them if we simply take care of them. We can reverse years of damage to our bodies by deciding to raise our standards for ourselves, then living differently. Old wounds heal, injuries repair, and the whole system improves with just a few changes in what we put into our bodies and how we move them.

Think about how you treat the car sitting in your driveway. Now think about how you treat your body. Which one gets the better treatment?

January 27

I can't believe I just ate the whole bag. I'll never do that again.
I'll start my diet first thing Monday.
I'm too sore to work out today.
I'm too tired to go running.
I want to lose weight, but I don't know how.
I don't have time to exercise.

Of all the people in the world you can lie to, the worst one is yourself. To trust anyone, you must first be able to trust yourself.

Lying to myself (particularly the "I'll start tomorrow" variety) is what got me to 371 pounds, diabetic, and with bum knees by the age of 30. Others haven't been so lucky. There are plenty of liars' graves in every cemetery. The ICU at the hospital is filled with liars, and there are scads of limbless liars wheeling about in wheelchairs. I know, because I was almost one of them.

Self lies also have a domino effect – one always leads to another. *I'll do something tomorrow* leads to *I'll start Monday* which takes you to *I'll just wait until the first of the month* and so on. They stack up one on top of the other and lead you down the path of destruction, where you're not living life, but simply existing. Or worse yet, waiting to die.

You cannot lie to yourself and have high self-esteem. Why would you, if you're a liar? Like I said, if you cannot trust yourself, you cannot trust anyone.

Admit to yourself what's making you unhappy – the source of your lies. Given the nature of my book, I'm going to assume here that it's your weight, size, fatness, or fitness. Admit that you're fat, and then decide to do something about it *immediately*.

I'm serious. Go do something now: throw out the cookies, take a walk, buy some exercise equipment, *something*. Face whatever fears you have. You might be afraid that people will laugh at you if they see you exercising. To hell with them! If they laugh, they laugh; it's their problem, not yours. I'm betting, though, that they won't. Most of the demons live entirely in your head, not in your neighborhood. It took me a long time to realize that people really didn't care about what I was doing when I was out in public. To them, I was just some other guy. A fat guy, sure, but the feeling of being a sideshow freak was all in my head.

The nice thing about being true to one's self is that it can have the same domino effect that lying does. One truth leads to another, which ultimately leads to a new trust and love for one's self. The accomplishments start piling up, the fat flies off, and your fitness level increases by leaps and bounds. What you're doing takes on its own life, and you wake up one day and find that you're a completely different person.

A person you love. A person you missed for many years. A person who can do anything. Isn't that what life's all about?

January 29

Most fat people got that way for a specific reason: they consumed more calories than they expended, over time. They either ate too much, moved too little, or both.

Into the life of every fat person comes pain, both mental and physical. Mental pain can include anguish over things like not being able to shop in the "normal" section of the clothing store, finding that you no longer fit in amusement park rides, or the looks of disgust you get (or imagine you get) from strangers. Physical pain from being fat comes from sources like your waist, because your pants are too tight, from your gut, which presses painfully into the table at any booth, or from your chest, where your heart is pounding madly after you climbed a flight of stairs.

Fat people know all about pain.

With pain can come anger – anger at the world for being so discriminatory, anger at your family for all their "helpful" comments that really hurt, and most of all anger with yourself, for letting yourself go to shit. That anger sits down deep, and it burns with a heat like no other, and in many (most, even) cases leads to diminished self-esteem, anti-social behavior, and self-loathing.

Fat people know all about anger and self-hatred.

I know a secret, though.

You don't have to do it any more if you don't want to. All you have to do is – are you ready for this? – let it go.

Forgive yourself.

Forgiveness doesn't mean forgetting what you did to get this way. It doesn't mean you're not responsible for the actions you took to get here. It means you acknowledge that you're not perfect, that you make (and have made) mistakes, and that you choose to love yourself and let them go. Regardless. What you did in the past, though it might have made you the person you are today, has absolutely no bearing on what you do in the future unless you let it, by sticking with the guilt, shame, blame, anger, and hatred. Let them go.

Forgive yourself and realize you've made mistakes. Accept yourself as what you were and as what you are, then resolve to have a different set of standards for yourself. Remember, you create your own reality, and you can make it whatever you want. Why not make it a good one?

February 2002

204 – 203 *pounds*

February 3

One of the stockers at the grocery store asked me yesterday if I'd lost weight. I said yes, and gave her the ballpark number because people love the numbers. She wanted to know how I did it and was shocked to find out I'd had no surgery. As it turns out one of her friends had the surgery and had dropped a goodly amount of weight. Her friend's biggest thrills now are being able to wear jeans again and being able to fit in the rides at Six Flags when they take the Girl Scout troop there.

I can relate to these thrills. The little things add up to one big reason to change. Whether it's fitting on the roller coasters or in a pair of jeans, or being able to go up stairs without panting like a racehorse, the little things combine and provide fuel for the desire necessary to transform your thinking and your life. The little things change your "I can't" into "I can," and they make your life metamorphose from just "getting by" to "living it to its fullest."

As with everything in life, what you do with regards to your health, body, and fitness is your choice. Do you choose to simply know the path, or do you choose to walk it?

February 9

How many times have you told yourself you're too fat to even bother trying to drop it? How many times have you told yourself that you're too old? Too out of shape? That you've failed too many times?

The only time it's too late to change yourself is when you're dead. Until then, you're simply making excuses or lying to yourself.

Was that harsh? Perhaps. Is it true? Definitely. You were made to excel, whether you have or not. Your body was made to move, to be active, no matter what you've done to it with food and sitting around. The earth is filled with a bounty of foods that can transform your body completely, though you've spent a lifetime poisoning yourself at the dinner table.

How many times have you gotten excited about changing yourself, only to never do it? If you're anything like I was, the answer to that question is "too many times to count." Why do we do that?

It has been said that the road to hell is paved with good intentions. We intend to change, we desire change, but we don't change. We procrastinate. We make excuses: "I'll start going to the gym when hunting season is over" or "I'll start eating healthier when my period ends, because there's no way I can control myself now."

We fail because we don't strike the iron while it's hot. We don't take immediate action toward achieving what we want. We decide to wait until tomorrow, or next week, or even next month. Then, sometime before the time we decided to start, our fire burns out because we're not stoking it. And we stay fat, again.

When I say immediate action, that's exactly what I mean. I mean right now. Make the decision, and do something right away – no matter how small – toward accomplishing what you want. It might be going for a walk or jog, or making a workout schedule, or throwing out some of the poison I mentioned earlier. Something. Don't just sit there.

If you're finding that these words are getting you excited, I'm wondering why you're still sitting there reading? Get up and go do something; the book's not going anywhere.

February 10

In the very beginning, I exercised because I knew I needed to. Over time, as my fitness improved somewhat, I grew to love exercise, believe it or not. As even more time passed, the idea of not exercising became foreign to me, resulting in my feeling "off" on days when I don't work out.

A habit was made, and I'm going to tentatively say that after almost two years (holy cow!) of doing it almost every day, I don't think I'll be suddenly changing this habit.

February 13

A stone that is not moving is an easy target for moss. A body that is not moving towards health and fitness is an easy target for obesity, heart disease, and diabetes. In the extreme case, a body that is not moving is dead.

What are you doing with your stone?

Have you set some health-related goals for yourself, and are you taking consistent action towards achieving whatever goals you've set? Are you living or dying? That's the one thing that gets to me when I see people who are in the station of life I was in just a couple of years ago. I remember being there, not really caring about how fat I was, and not living life at all. I was a big fat slug waiting to die. Until, that is, I realized that I really *was* going to die, and probably in the not too distant future.

And now – please forgive me if I cannot verbalize this properly; it's a very strong feeling within me – I wake up every day with the realization that this is it, that there's only one shot at this life and I can either enjoy the ride and live it to its fullest and to my highest potential or I can screw it up and go back to being that fat guy who was eating his way to four hundred pounds.

I'd rather not screw it up. If there's one thing I'm passionate about these days, it is that. The notion of getting the most life has to offer so that when I'm old and dying, I can look back and know beyond the shadow of a doubt that I have no regrets. I'll know that I'm not some unmoving rock that just sat there throughout life, packing on layer after layer of moss, but that I rolled like a son-of-a-bitch, and enjoyed every second of it.

February 21

Many times, super-sized people look at where they are compared to where they want to be, and are overwhelmed by the sheer magnitude of the task they perceive before them. Often, people have asked me how I could have ever started, knowing I needed to drop close to two hundred pounds of fat from my body. Regularly, fat people talk about this overwhelm and decide to break their dream into smaller – more manageable, to them – pieces, of five or ten pounds at a time.

There's an old saying I really like: "if you can dream it, you can achieve it." We all hold within us a great and awesome power: the power to dream up fantastic things for ourselves. We also have the ability within us to make those dreams into realities, but fear holds us back.

We've failed so many times; we don't want to fail again. We wonder if people will still like us. We worry about the new life waiting, because it's so foreign to us. We fear, and we limit ourselves. Use your power. Dream big, and achieve big. If nothing else, I'm proof that you can set your mind to something then go about accomplishing it, no matter what. Big dreams are powerful things indeed. Don't limit yourself with a little dream, reach inside and come up with something big. Then make it happen.

February 23

Someone's watching you.

Not Santa Claus.

Not Jesus.

Not God.

Your spouse is watching you.

Your kids are watching you.

Your friends are watching you.

Your neighbors are watching you.

Your co-workers are watching you.

The people at church are watching you, as well as all the people in whatever social groups you may belong.

Why are they watching you?

Your first instinct – based on the words of some cruel and uncaring person, perhaps – might be to think they're watching you just to see you fail, because you've failed so many times.

They're not.

You might think they're watching you to judge you. To see if you're going to "slip" or eat something you "shouldn't" have. Possibly, but most likely not. They're watching you to see what you'll do, because they believe in you. They like – love, in many cases – you. They respect you.

Are there assholes? Yes, of course. Like the poor, the assholes will always be with us. But, no matter what you think, most people aren't assholes. Most people are pretty good, and want good things to come not only to themselves but to those around them.

And so they watch you for guidance. They watch the example you lead in life, in many regards. Given the nature of this book, I'm speaking about your choices relating to your health, obviously, but they're watching you for many other things.

What kind of example are you setting for them? Are you true to yourself? Do you feed your body with the high-octane fuel it deserves, or do you regularly fill it with garbage? Do you work your body, reaching new heights of strength and movement, or do you sit and atrophy?

Give them something to look at.

February 26

Several years ago, when I was teaching my daughter how to ride a bike, we went to a local church parking lot for her to practice. The lot was small, as was the church, and there was a single streetlight pole at one side of the lot. I was too fat to run behind her holding the seat of the bike, but I was strong enough to hold her in place and give her a good push to start the bike moving at a fast enough clip so she could stay balanced. The first time I pushed her across the lot, she rode fairly well, staying balanced but not really pedaling.

But she noticed the streetlight pole as she ended that first ride.

"What if I run into the pole?" she asked, wheeling the bike back across the parking lot toward me.

"Don't worry, you're not going to. You're not going anywhere near it," I replied.

Au contraire.

The very next time I pushed her, the bike veered like a homing pigeon and she rode it straight into the pole, which was only pole in the entire parking lot. She fell, of course, and squalled loudly though she was merely scared and not injured. We went home then, and she was too scared to try bike riding again for about three more years, and only then because her grandpa pushed her into trying. As a result of what she focused on that day – the pole – she drove herself into it, and as a result of that, the fear she focused on kept her from trying again for several years.

If you aren't happy with the person you are, focus on the person you want to be. Your mind will automatically start to transform you into that person. Overnight? No. Over time? Yes, as long as you maintain your focus.

The goal is not to focus on how "perfect" you've been, or to obsess over some number on a scale, but to live consistently as the person you want to be. If you make a mistake – and you are human – get over it. Don't get paralyzed by fear and give up. Pick yourself up, dust off your behind, and renew your focus. It's really that easy. Don't get caught up in the "what if" questions, because they serve no purpose beyond breeding fear.

February 28

Scientists just announced that a diet high in processed meats can increase the risk of developing adult-onset diabetes in men. Just in case you need another reason to stop eating garbage.

March – August 2002

203 – 200 pounds

March 4

I've been asked several times recently about the idea of a "free day," where you set aside a certain amount of time each week – be it a meal, two meals, or an entire day – and anything goes with regards to eating. The theory is this: you cannot screw yourself up in a single day, and a free day makes mid-week cravings easier to deal with because you know that you can have anything you desire – healthy or not – on your free day.

Initially, I was mostly ambivalent toward the notion (which was popularized in the book *Body-for-Life*, by Bill Phillips), with a slight leaning towards not liking it because it was a succession of free days that got me to the point where I weighed almost 400 pounds. Additionally, I saw people who follow the *Body-for-Life* program tend to obsess over upcoming free days, and that sparked a slight concern that such activities could lead back to being super-fat.

I decided to test the idea of a free day for myself, so that I could speak more authoritatively about it, rather than proclaiming my judgment without ever having actually tried it. I now present you with the results of The Great Free Day Experiment of 2002.

For three Fridays running, I've taken "free days." On those Fridays, I determined to eat whatever my heart might possibly desire, whether it was healthy or not. Have I missed certain foods over the last almost two years? A little, perhaps. I like the way I feel a lot more than I liked any of the foods I once ate regularly but every once in a while I do get a hankering for some real garbage. This is just what the free day is for.

My first free day, three weeks ago, I got up and did my normal weight/cardio routine. After my workout, I had my usual protein shake, and followed over the day with a normal breakfast and a normal lunch. At dinnertime, however, we went out for Mexican and I had a huge amount of chips and salsa, and steak fajitas with guacamole and sour cream. After dinner, I came home and later had two big bowls of Cheerios with sugar, and followed that up with two cream-filled-chocolate-covered doughnuts Robyn picked up for me when she went to get some ice cream for herself and our daughter.

When Monday morning rolled around, the scale showed a pound gone from the week before. Note that even if the number had been up, it wouldn't have been important, because you cannot really do damage to yourself in one day's eating. Your body simply cannot handle that kind of an inflow of calories, and you pass most of them out via normal elimination.

The next Friday, I decided to up the stakes, to prove a point. A workout once again fell on this day, so I had my usual post-workout shake. At work I had a usual breakfast then followed it with four chocolate-covered doughnuts (apparently I'd been craving the doughnuts and didn't know it). I ate a normal lunch, then picked up five fried chicken fingers, a box of pizza rolls, a box of fried cheese, and half a pecan pie from the grocery store for dinner. I ate it all, plus a piece of the pizza Robyn got for herself and our daughter, as well as a couple of candy bars.

I weighed another pound less the following Monday.

The third Friday, this past one, was a total crap-fest. That day coincided with a no-workout day, so there was no shake. Instead, I had a big bowl of cereal, a peanut butter egg, and a candy bar. On the way to work, I bought three chocolate-covered doughnuts, a blueberry-filled doughnut, and a cream-filled-chocolate-covered doughnut.

And that was breakfast.

For a midmorning snack, I had a box of pizza rolls. Lunch was red beans and rice I'd brought from home, followed by a box of fried cheese. Dinner was five corndogs and another box of fried cheese. Dessert was an entire pecan pie save the single small piece I gave my daughter. Once again, I weighed a pound less this morning. I weigh 202 pounds, down three pounds over the three weeks I experimented with the free day concept.

There were a couple of caveats to this whole experiment, however. First, remember that I work out intensely very regularly. I cannot say a free day will work if you're not doing the same. Second, I ate *very* clean for the other six days of the week: none of my normal grabbing a small snack if I got hungry between meals. If I got hungry between meals on any day except Friday, I stayed hungry until the next meal.

Will a free day work for you? I don't know, but you might want to give it a try if you find yourself prone to cravings. Will I continue to use Friday as a free day? Yes, but not nearly to the extent that I did during the experiment. Friday was already a "sort of" free day, because I'd have a bite of a candy bar, or a couple of cookies that day anyway, since it's Robyn's free day.

There was another interesting side effect of going to town on so much crappy food: without fail, at the end of each Friday I was thankful it was over, and was looking forward to getting up the next morning to eat good healthful foods again.

March 9

I've noticed that though my weight and body fat continue to decrease, I'm still chunky.

Not because I don't have big enough muscles.

Not because I still perceive myself as a fat guy.

I'm a large man wearing an extra-extra-large suit of skin.

I've mentioned before that I have a little loose skin, but not much. Relative to many people I've encountered that's true. I don't have a big apron; I have a wrinkly belly and big saggy man-boobs. I have a paunch, and a low roll of skin at my waistline. If I'm lying on my back at night and I shift, I'll usually have some skin roll up and pinch under me because it's so loose. Pretty much anywhere on my torso below my chest (front and back) I can grab up handfuls of skin.

The problem is, as Fred gets smaller, Fred's skin doesn't. I would never dare to take my shirt off in public, nor would I wear a skintight shirt, because my skin looks like fat when it's packed in. I can fold off an 8- or 10-inch section of stomach skin with no problem now.

There are two things right now that are vying for first place on my hate-o-meter. One is that if I pull the skin tight, anywhere, I can see rippling muscles. For example, if I grab a double handful of belly skin and pull it tight, I can count the cans in my six-pack. My pectorals are awesome, wide and flaring, but two big flaps of boob skin dangle below them. My back muscles give me an awesome v-shape but they're covered by hanging flaps of skin on my sides.

There's not much that sucks as much as getting glimpses of an awesome body when you manipulate the skin, and then having it look all pudgy and flabby when you let the skin go back to its normal place. Or being able to feel bulging and rippling muscles, only to not be able to see them because of the skin.

The other thing high on the hate-o-meter is having part of my body over which I have no control. I'm not known for my delicacy with words, so I'm going to shoot straight from the hip here. The thing that tipped me over the edge with regards to this skin was being in a rather compromising position with my wife and making the mistake of looking down my body.

Gravity can do evil things with loose skin when you're in a position very similar to doing pushups. Beautiful pectorals, flexed from supporting my weight, then two big long pointy skin sacks. Man-boobs. There's a clear line of demarcation between the pectoral muscle and the skin sack, like the line dividing North and South Korea. I have my very own axis of evil, right on my chest.

But the boobs aren't the worst part, not even close. The worst part is my stomach, which, not being held in place by my abs, hangs down almost a foot. It's just a big empty sack, swinging from side to side. It's not there when I'm standing, you know, because I can use my abs somewhat to hold it in place. But, I found that if I relax my abs while standing straight, my gut sack droops and flops around limply. I don't like this one bit.

While I've contended all along that dropping weight is easy – and I still believe that – I've also contended that life changes require effort. In the case of building up some decent muscles, it takes some pretty serious effort.

Am I angry? Yes, a little. I've busted my butt in the gym to build the decent muscles I just mentioned, and I cannot see a lot of them because of this damn skin. The thing that makes me most angry is the fact that I'm ashamed (and on a side note, I am completely aware that the ashamedness is simply a choice I make) to take my shirt off in public. For my entire adult life, any time I was swimming with people other than Robyn and our daughter, I've worn a shirt. Then, I thought I was too fat. Now, I'm too saggy and loose, for lack of better words.

I'm unhappy with the situation, but I do know a way to help remedy it should I choose to.

This past Thursday, I visited another plastic surgeon. This experience was 100% different from the last. This man was *much* more professional, listened to my complaints, and told me several things. He can remedy my man-boobs, he said. He can remove the extra skin there, and make my chest look like a normal man's. And my pectorals will show.

On my stomach, he can do basically the same thing: cutting me from hip to hip, leaving my belly button on a little stalk, then removing a football-shaped piece of skin roughly 12 or 14 inches wide at its widest point.

Without doing anything to my abs.

"The other surgeon I talked to was insistent on stitching up my abs," I commented.

"Your abs are great," he said, "They're very tight. If they were loose, maybe, but yours aren't."

There was something else, too.

"The other surgeon wanted to liposuction me everywhere, to contour me. Is that necessary?" I asked.

"No," he said, simply, "there's nothing in there to liposuction. It's just skin."

There's nothing in there to liposuction. It's gone. For good.

If I were to get the surgery it would take about four hours and I could go home that day. I could be exercising in just over a week, he told me, and doing resistance training in two. Not six weeks like with the first doctor, because this option is, while serious, much less intrusive than liposuction and muscle-stitching.

Will I do it? I don't know. I'm still mulling it over. It's very tempting, the thought of running around in a muscle shirt or shirtless, and not worrying about flopping and flapping and jiggling. It's also very scary, because I've never had surgery before, never been under the knife. And, of course, the question arises in my mind as to whether or not this whole issue is worth ten thousand dollars.

March 16

I've decided – after months of saying I wasn't going to, and a goodly amount of time mulling it over – to have my excess skin removed by a surgeon in the near future.

If I were to ask you what the most important "secret" to transforming your body is, what would you tell me?

Diet? Maybe.

Exercise? Maybe.

I want to suggest something different, something that is far more important that what you eat or how you move. Don't get me wrong, both of those are very important – I cannot imagine much of a transformation where you still eat crap food all the time and never get physical – but there's one more tiny little thing that pulls it all together, and this tiny little thing is the key.

Consistency.

Consistency keeps you working out regularly, even if you miss the occasional day. Consistency keeps you generally choosing good fuel sources for your body, even if you sometimes choose the not so good. It's what separates the successes from the failures, because consistent people realize that one indiscretion neither ends the world nor undoes months of changes.

March 18

Ah, Monday.

I rolled out of the bed at a couple of minutes past four, ready to go downstairs and do my upper body weightlifting workout. It was a little chilly in the garage, but warmer than it had been for quite some time. I knew that by the end of a couple of sets of chest presses I'd be warmed up, so I didn't put on my winter underwear, opting instead to wear nothing more than my boxer briefs and a t-shirt.

Outside, rain fell practically sideways, driven into the garage door like liquid nails by the moaning wind. Lightning flashed from time to time, and I heard low thunder in the distance.

My lifting was without special incident, and as it drew to an end my mind turned to cardiovascular training.

"True," I said to myself, "but the alternatives are worse. I could skip cardio, I could ride the stationary bike, or I could do some kickboxing with Billy Blanks."

All of which sparked not a smidgen of interest, so I decided to brave the rain.

When my weight routine was over, I stripped out of my boxer briefs and put on some running shorts. There's just something cool about running in running shorts with no underwear, as long as you don't get hit by a car or accidentally expose yourself to other runners.

I wrapped the garage door opener in Glad wrap and put it in my pocket, hung my identification tag around my neck, and set off down the driveway at my ploddingly slow pace. The rain was cold, pricking my exposed skin and making me shiver. I warmed up quickly, however, since the outdoor temperature was fairly moderate. Like my weightlifting, my run was without special incident.

I got wet. Very wet. Soaked. I returned to my house cold and dripping. Water was in my eyes, squelching in my shoes, and my t-shirt clung to me like a second skin. As soon as the garage door closed behind me, I stripped off my wet clothes and looked for a towel with which to dry. There were two: one that we normally use as a pad for squats hanging on the Smith machine, and one in the corner of the garage, sitting on the ground nicely folded. I decided to use the latter, walked across the garage, and picked it up, shaking it open and popping it like a whip a couple of times to make sure there was no extra dirt on it.

I took a deep breath and hung the towel over my head. It covered my head completely and hung to my belly button in the front and almost to my butt in the back. Vigorously I attacked my wet hair, rubbing the towel over my head repeatedly. I wiped my face with the towel, dried my cheeks and inside my ears. I blotted my lips dry with the towel then wiped down my neck, arms, and chest.

It wasn't until I was exuberantly wiping my groin with the towel that I noticed it, enveloping me like a foul yellow cloud.

One of the cats had peed on the towel.

March 20

Today, the rubber met the road. I called the plastic surgeon to find out how soon he could perform the operation. Next Thursday morning is open. It turns out I'm not the big fearless man I thought I was.

I got nervous at the thought of surgery for something that's not life threatening. *Surely other people have had this done and posted stories about it online*, my mind said, leading me to start a search on a search engine. Which led me to finding numerous people's personal stories about skin removal surgery. With the exception of one story, they all had:

- Gallons and gallons of nastiness draining out of them, for weeks. I expected draining, but only for a few days.
- Infections. Lots of infections. Stinky, smelly, pus-laden, oozing infections.
- Pain. For weeks and weeks, not the few days I expected.
- Wounds that reopened on their own – usually because the internal pressure from dead and rotting blood building up in the abdominal cavity.
- A couple of them also had some *necrosis*, a lovely side effect where your skin dies and starts rotting. In many cases this skin that dies is your belly button, which turns black.

In the interests of fairness, let me also point out that in every single case, these people were much larger than me, had much more loose skin and, if I may be vain, were in much worse physical shape than I am. Also, without exception, every single one had had weight-loss surgery previously.

But still, those are some nasty complications for something that's not life-threatening.

Thus, I waffled. Again.

I've seen both sides of the issue, from the surgeon's rosy view to the not-so-pretty view of people who've been through it, and I must say, I'm pretty convinced I really can live with the skin I've got, if it means no drains, no infections, no pain, and no oozing and spontaneous re-openings. Put me in a fight or flight situation (or perceived one) and I will take flight every single time.

Call me Waffle Man; no one has to live my life but me.

March 23

As much as I enjoy the food I have on free day, by the time I go to bed, I'm more than ready for my normal "clean" food. When your body gets used to the primo fuel, crappy food – though it may taste good going down – just doesn't make the engine run right, and the engine's begging for the good stuff when free day ends. I get heartburn at night, and I have heartburn and acidic burps during my Saturday morning run.

My point is this: if you have troubles eating clean, consider a free day occasionally. It might be once a week, it might be once a month. Let yourself eat what you want, and you'll find that your body begs for the healthy stuff when it's all over.

April 5

Once again, I've changed my mind about having the skin removal surgery. I cannot stand the loose skin any more. I'm scheduled to go in on April 10 at 7:00 am, and should be home by 3:00 or 4:00 that afternoon. The plastic surgeon is going to take me in, knock me out, and cut me open, making me tight where I am loose.

He assures me I should have none of the horrific side effects I'm concerned about, because I'm such good shape and good health. He also told me – because I asked – that he's never lost anyone on the operating table.

I trust him, and I cannot wait to see the new tighter Fred.

April 12

I had my skin removal surgery two days ago, and everything went perfectly. I was in surgery by 9:00 am and out by about 1:00. My plastic surgeon removed less than three pounds of skin and fat from my body. That's right, I said fat. He *tried* to do liposuction on me in both my sides and in my chest, but only managed to get about a cup of fat altogether. After the surgery he told me he got as much as he could, but there just wasn't any there to get. The vast majority of what he took from me was extra skin, and though it's too soon to tell yet what the final result will be, I'm already happy because everything's so *tight* now. I'll be able to tell more when some of the swelling goes down.

I'm tired and a little sore right now, but not terribly. I've already stopped taking the pain pills he gave me. Mostly the pain in my chest and abdomen is about as bad as when I change my weightlifting routine. By far the worst pain of the surgery was the removal of the catheter, which was done *after* I woke up. That's something I hope to never go through again.

April 14

Just when I thought nothing interesting could happen for me to write about while I recuperate, I went and fell down the stairs yesterday. I was heading downstairs to get more coffee when it happened. I was wearing my bright red Hershey Kiss sleep pants, an XXXXXL shirt from my fattest days, and my blue slippers. In one hand I carried my super-sized coffee mug – the one that's so big a whole pot won't even fill it twice. Robyn was behind me on the landing, looking for cleaning supplies in the closet.

I was on the second step – *the second step*, for God's sake – when my foot landed and skipped off that step and loudly down to the next one, causing a big thump. I flailed my left hand, the one with the not-quite-empty coffee mug wildly, spilling none, and slammed my empty right hand into the banister. Robyn gasped, as she is prone to helpfully do in certain situations.

"I guess I don't need to wear my slippers on the stairs, huh?" I said, laughing.

"Be careful, baby!" she admonished from within the closet, "You could really hurt yourself, in your condition."

I took the next step, this time with the other foot, and did it again, only this time my foot skipped down three stairs – *bambambam* – like I was skiing and I went down onto my ass and started bumping merrily along.

Robyn screamed loudly, but not helpfully, and ran to the top of the stairs clutching a bottle of bleach. Again I flailed my arms wildly, and again I managed to catch a banister before I'd gone too terribly far. And again, I spilled no coffee at all.

I sat there for a moment, unable to get up because I was laughing so hard. My wife failed to see the humor in the situation, given my current state of disrepair, but I was cackling like a fool at my inability to navigate a staircase. One of our cats ran up the stairs chirping, possibly in an attempt to hurl her rather portly body into my path to stop me should I fall again. Danielle ran out of her room to stare at me.

After a few minutes I was able to finish my trek down the stairs for more coffee, which I ultimately ended up not drinking because I'd gotten so hot from laughing so hard. Robyn finally saw the humor in the whole situation and laughed with me, and we spent the better part of the day joking about the great fall of '02.

I did, however, learn a very important lesson yesterday: they're called "slippers" for a reason.

April 15

I had to go see the plastic surgeon today for a follow-up to my skin removal surgery, and he told me something surprising. Something humorous.

"Go to Sears or JC Penney," he said, "and buy a girdle."

"A girdle?" I asked, blinking at him, "Like women wear?"

"Yup," he told me, "like women wear."

At the mall, Robyn and I went into JC Penney and spent several minutes looking for the unmentionables before finally deciding they must be on the second floor. That's exactly where we found them, right next to the very crowded customer service area. Fortunately, the bras and panties – neither of which I needed, but would probably look good in – occupied the space right next to the counter and the customers, while the girdles ("body shapers" they're called in today's politically correct world, it seems) were off in a dingy little corner by themselves.

We walked over, Robyn normally and me slowly shuffling like an old man. I felt like I needed to be wearing an overcoat with nothing on underneath. While she looked through the girdles, I studiously counted ceiling tiles and tried to make myself invisible. Unfortunately, I think I only succeeded in looking conspicuous. That's how it felt, at least.

Women, I found when Robyn started trying to put girdles on me in the store, are seriously skinny compared to men. The girdle sized XL didn't even make it across my ass, and I don't have a big ass. The XXL, which was the largest size they had, crossed my ass and made it to my sides, but that's it. I suggested we go to Lane Bryant, a store for more ample-sized women.

The trip down the mall was interminable. For the first time ever, I had to tell Robyn to slow down. Usually she's telling me to because I have longer legs and therefore a longer stride. Plus, I tend to always be in a hurry when I'm walking because I want to be wherever I'm going.

We finally made it to Lane Bryant and went inside. Fortunately, there were only a couple of customers so I figured my embarrassment would be kept to an absolute minimum. As is par for these things, I figured wrong. We couldn't find the corset-type girdles, which is what I wanted. We could only find the panty-type girdles, so I had to go find a salesperson to give us some assistance while Robyn continued to look.

"Excuse me," I said to the young girl behind the counter. She looked up expectantly, and my mind went totally blank. I had no idea how to ask what I needed to ask, so I babbled.

"I just had some surgery," I said quickly, "and I need to get a girdle to compress my abdomen so the doctor doesn't have to cut me back open and drain me with a rubber tube but all we can find is the kind of girdles that have the panty parts attached and I figure those squeeze everything and being a guy there are certain parts I don't really want to have squeezed all the time."

She blinked at me.

"Heh," I said.

"I don't know," she finally said, slyly, "you might enjoy it!"

Just what I needed, a sassy clerk. We walked back over to where Robyn was looking at the panty-girdles and the clerk told us that those were the only kind the store carries.

"Can I cut the crotch out of it?" I asked, "Cause I'm a man, and there's just certain things I don't want squeezed, you know."

"I guess you can," she replied, "but I still think you ought to try it. You might like it."

"I've got drains coming out down there, and it would hurt too much to have the area squeezed. Other than that, you're probably right, I *would* enjoy it."

I realized how I sounded.

"Jeez, I'm sorry," I said, "that's probably more than you wanted to know. I'm probably freaking you out with all this talk about my surgery."

"Oh, no, that's fine," she said, "I've seen it all. We have a lot of drag queens in here and they're a lot crazier than you."

"I'M NOT A DRAG QUEEN!" I practically shouted, turning red because I felt like a drag queen in the Lane Bryant looking at silky girdles.

"I know you're not," she said, not looking she believed herself.

We ultimately decided to get one of the sexy, sensual – I kid you not, it says that on the label – girdles for me to wear, thus bringing about an eternal discussion between my wife and the clerk about what size I might wear. Because there's no rational relationship between women's sizes and women's measurements, me knowing my waist size was no help at all. Finally, they decided I'd probably be an 18/20, whatever that is. I'm not sure if I should feel fat or not. The clerk and I went to the counter so I could pay for my girdle.

"I think you'll be happy with this," she said, walking around another employee who was on the telephone, "I wear these myself every day and love them."

I considered asking her if I could see, but I thought that might be in poor taste.

"I hope it works well too," I said, "If it does, I'll send my wife back down to get me a couple more."

The employee on the telephone turned around to stare at me, like I was some kind of freakish drag queen.

May 18

It's official, five weeks after my surgery: my man-boobs have mostly vanished and my belly is almost perfectly flat. I can no longer grab double handfuls of skin around my waist and stretch them out six inches. As a matter of fact, all I can pinch up is the tiniest little bit of skin, because I think the surgeon climbed up on the operating table with me and *leaned* into it to pull my skin tight.

The whole thing was a piece of cake. Little pain, lots of pleasure – I look at myself a lot more now, and with pride instead of disgust at my droopy skin. No complications: no rotting skin, no seromas, no ruptured incisions, and my scars are perfectly flat. My abdominal scar is so low it's hidden by underwear. Obviously the chest scars are more visible, but I still look good in a tight shirt.

There's still a little swelling, and I puff up during the day because fluid collects above the waist incision. According to my surgeon, the operation disrupted all the pathways that the lymphatic serum used when moving around the area, so it collects temporarily during the day. It vanishes at night, and it swells a little less each day. If I follow the normal pattern, within another month or two it'll be gone completely. And lest you think it's bad swelling, it is not; Robyn cannot tell a difference when she looks at me, but I can see it. Of course, I look at me more than anyone else does.

The one downside to everything is that I got hepatitis A shortly after the surgery. Not as a result of the surgery and not from the hospital, because the incubation period wasn't really long enough. Most likely I came into contact with it a couple of weeks before the surgery, and only developed it because my immune system was weakened from the operation. Even so, I was only feeling bad enough to skip working out for less than a week. I'm almost completely back to normal from that; I had my liver function tested Thursday and most of the readings are only slightly elevated now instead of being through the roof like when I was first diagnosed.

Speaking of working out, I was walking 2.5 miles a day less than ten days after my surgery, and lifting weights again right at the two-week mark. The hepatitis nixed that for a little while, but I'm back to lifting four days a week and walk-jogging six, just like before the surgery. I'm still not back to my full strength but I'm getting stronger every day, which is good.

On the weight front, things are a little funny. On surgery morning, I weighed in at 203.5. Shortly after surgery, the swelling shot me up to about 220 before it started coming back down. Weighing became a game, because it was fun to watch things change around so much each day. About ten days back I rolled across 200, and in the last week it slid on down to 196. I'm still eating the same, but if I get to 190, I guess I'm going to start eating more. My guess is that I was really dropping the weight all along after the surgery, but the swelling covered it up until just recently.

In any case, it's odd to be back to the days where I'm dropping 3 or 4 pounds a week, but it's kind of cool to have hit the 175-pounds-gone mark, despite my beliefs on the non-importance of such things as scale weight.

July 16

I've been great. My hepatitis is completely gone, and my health is back 100% from the surgery, too. I'm lifting weights three days a week and running – no more walk-jogging, pure running now – three miles also three days a week, alternating with the weightlifting days. I still take Sundays off.

On the physical side, my weight bounces around between 195 and 198 pounds, depending on all the various factors that affect one's weight on a daily basis. I still eat junk food on Fridays, though generally it's more or less just a big evening meal and some sweets before bed, instead of a whole day of eating crap. The all-junk days were just making me feel sluggish and gross the whole weekend, so I cut them back.

It's all about the fuel, remember?

August 21

In my current weightlifting routine, I do a four-week endurance building cycle of low weights with high reps, a four-week size-building cycle of heavy weights with medium reps, and a total butt-kicking four-week strength building cycle of ultra-heavy weights at very low reps per set. After a complete 12-week rotation I take a week off to recover, walking instead of running and lifting little or no weights.

I'm currently in one of these weeks off, and decided to do one of my wife's "Firm" videos because the thought of walking – despite the enjoyable audio book I'm listening to – had no appeal at all to me. I watch my wife's videos while I lift weights, and they look pretty simple to do, even though my wife tells me otherwise. The video I selected is called "Maximum Body Shaping" and is taught by Master Instructor Tracie Long. For my workout, I chose a set of 5-pound dumbbells, a set of 10-pound dumbbells, and a set of 20-pound dumbbells. I am, after all, in top physical shape now and such light weights would be perfect for this simple little workout.

I popped the video into the VCR and stepped back from the television. My weights were arranged across the floor in front of me, and all the benches and whatnot in the gym were moved aside to give me plenty of room to work out. The Fanny Lifter™, a glorified step that came with the "Firm" videos, was off to my right.

The commercials advertising other "Firm" videos played, and then there she was: Master Instructor Tracie Long. She looked friendly and perky and happy in her little white shirt and black shorts, standing there in front of the rest of her class. She wanted to start out with a nice warm up so we began marching together.

We marched for about 30 seconds, then Master Instructor Tracie Long transformed before my eyes, from Master Instructor to Rockette. She began kicking her legs in all directions – left, right, forward, and backwards – over her head every single time. She jumped. She spun. She danced madly, a whirling dervish on the screen. The rest of the group kept perfect step with her throughout the mad movements.

The rest of the group except for me, that is.

I watched stupidly from my position in front of the television, feeling like the little fat kid that no one would play with because he couldn't keep up. *The heck with her,* I thought to myself, *these dance moves are for women and girly-men.* I waited patiently for the weightlifting part, trying to keep up with some of the easier dance moves but mostly just marching in place with the occasional half-hearted kick.

After what felt like twenty minutes of the cardio-kick-jump-dancing, it was time for a little stretching. Master Instructor Tracie Long instructed me to flip my foot back and catch it with my hand behind my butt in the classic quadriceps stretch. No problem. Then she stood, perfectly immobile and zen-like, holding the stretch. I stood as immobile as possible as long as I could before hopping frantically around the garage on one leg in a desperate attempt to maintain my balance. I tripped over the Fanny Lifter™ and almost fell down, but was fortunately able to catch myself with my hip and shoulder on the home gym. Master Instructor Tracie Long stared at me, inscrutable.

Finally, she put her leg down and stretched her other quadriceps. I stretched mine too, but only for about ten percent of the time in which she did hers. By holding my chin-up bar I managed to not fall down this time. Master Instructor Tracie Long took us through some more stretches, and I mostly kept up. The warm-up ended, and it was time for the *real* workout. I was already sweating profusely and breathing hard. Master Instructor Tracie Long, along with the entire rest of the class, appeared to be just as fresh as when the tape started.

I grabbed my heavy weights, at her instruction, to do squats. Lots of squats. Squats, followed by pushups. *Slow* pushups, where you hold yourself with your chest one inch off the ground for ten seconds at a time. We did a long and protracted set of these pushups, and then we did more squats. After the squats? We did more pushups, of course. During the second set of pushups I had to switch from military-style (on my toes) to kiddie-style (on my knees) because I was afraid I was going to collapse.

Master Inquisitor Torquemada Long and the rest of the priests popped right up for some more weight routines. Unfortunately I cannot remember what they did next, because I was lying on the ground through it, trying to catch my breath.

When I was able to breathe normally again, I got up just in time to do one-arm rows, which I did with my left arm. Biceps curls, overhead presses, upright rows, and roughly seven thousand lunges done holding a broomstick followed the rows. When it was time to repeat the entire sequence with the right side, I think I got confused and did the left again. I'm not sure, because I was hallucinating by then from a lack of oxygen.

We did plyometric jumps until my knees ached, then this strange combination of stepping up on the Fanny Lifter™, tapping one foot or the other, and stepping down gracefully (well, Master Inquisitor Torquemada Long was graceful; I was more like Willard in *Footloose*) only to repeat the maneuver with the other foot. This lasted easily an hour, then it was time for some more upper body work so the Wicked Witch of the West led us through military presses, deltoid raises for all three heads of the muscle, triceps kickbacks, and more biceps curls for good measure. I mostly kept up, except for when I had to stop and take drags off the oxygen tank and mop sweat off my face with a big towel. Evil Witch Tracie and the rest of the class had not yet broken a sweat.

Next came more lunges, both forwards and backwards. Everyone seemed to love them even though they did them for fifteen minutes. I sat on the Fanny Lifter™ and watched them.

After the lunges and dips, she decided to round things out with a few more sets of squats. I was able to do the first few sets, sort of. By now my squats were more mental than physical. Instead of going until my thighs were parallel to the floor, I lowered myself until they were parallel with the wall. I looked at the time counter on the tape and noted that I'd only been working out for about 35 minutes total. I had a brief second to wonder if I'd slipped into a time differential before she announced it was time for abdominal work.

I took a moment to wipe more sweat off my body and see that she and the rest of her demons were still completely sweat free, then I made myself supine for the crunches. The crunches were actually fun. The rest of the abdominal workout was not. I spent most of it alternately crying and praying for a swift death. I wished for the Second Coming. I shot hate rays from my eyes to the television, but she was able to easily deflect them. Her eyes glowed red as she cackled at my suffering.

And then, the most magical moment of the whole video came.

"We're almost done," she said, fire and brimstone falling from her mouth as she spoke, "Just a little more chest work."

Over the course of my life I have learned, through a great deal of time spent studying the Bible, that Satan is the father of lies. This morning, I met the mother.

By no stretch of my fevered imagination could the infinity of flyes, pullovers, and French presses we did be called "a little chest work." Granted, I was delirious by this point, but I drifted into lucidity a few times and every time I did, I was still working my chest. Just before I passed out from exhaustion she ended it, and decreed it was time to stretch.

I lay on the floor in a heap, panting and sweating, and watched them stretch. By the time they were finished, I was able to climb slowly to my feet and walk shakily over to the VCR to hit the stop button.

I think I'll try the advanced tape tomorrow.

August 31

Is your life everything you want it to be? Are you at the fitness level where you can do more than you'd ever want without getting tired? Are you excited every morning when you get out of bed, because it's a new day waiting to be filled with vibrant living? Can you outrun, outplay, and out-chase your children? If you answered no to any (or all) of these, it's okay. I'm here to tell you the good news.

You have some magic in you. You might not know about it yet, but it's there. The magic that can transform you from what you are now to everything you ever dreamed you could be – and more. All you have to do is use it. Make a commitment to yourself to expend some effort each day to bettering yourself. I've talked a lot about "worth" over the last couple of years, and this time is no different. Nothing in this world is as valuable as you are, and nothing can be worth more to you than yourself. Yes, your children are valuable and your spouse is valuable, but if you're not your best you cannot give your best to them. Use the magic you have in you, and set a new standard for yourself. Decide that you're in charge of you – not food, not the television, you.

Get rid of the garbage in your kitchen. If you believe we are what we eat, then I must ask you this: do you want to be an over-processed pile of chemicals, artificial colors and flavors, and trans-fatty acids? Do you want to live in the house that pizza built? You know what's healthy, what your body craves and needs.

Get off the couch. You don't have to be able to run a marathon or dead-lift 1000 pounds to be in shape, all you have to do is move. Find the joy of playing with your children, romping through the sprinklers or walking in the woods. Learn from them – they're nothing but bundles of energy.

Above all, quit trying to be perfect. You aren't. I'm not. No one is. You cannot ever be perfect, no matter how hard you try, but you know what? You can always be a little better today than you were yesterday.

Try it, and create the life of your dreams.

Acknowledgements

Thanks to:

Sarah Cypher, the Threepenny Editor, for her invaluable work in editing and copywriting. If you like what you read herein, it is because of her; if you do not, it is because of me.

Marie Gilbert, for designing the interior layout and putting up with my neurotic behavior over it.

Mike Cox of Alpha Advertising, for doing such a bang-up job on the cover.

The people at Vaughan Printing, who created the book you now hold.

The fine folks at Three Toes Publishing, for their wonderful job at book production.

My wife and love of my life Robyn, for believing in me when no one else did.

All the readers of my web sites, who came along for the ride from chunk to hunk.

Finally, to The Learning Channel, for having the right show on at the right time.

About the Author: Fred Anderson lives in Alabama with his wife Robyn, their daughter Danielle, and five ornery and cantankerous cats. He works as a software engineer during the day, and spends his nights surfing online and reading. Fred can be visited online at http://www.chunktohunk.com, or emailed at fred@chunktohunk.com